NURSING DEVELOPMENT UNITS
A Force for Change

NURSING DEVELOPMENT UNITS

UNITS

A Force for Change

Edited by

Jane Salvage RN BA MSc
Regional Adviser for Nursing and Midwifery, Regional Office for
Europe, World Health Organization

and

Stephen G Wright RN RNT DipN DANS MSc FRCN MBE
Director, The European Nursing Development Agency (TENDA)
and Visiting Professor of Nursing, University of Southampton

SCUTARI PRESS
London

© Scutari Press, 1995
Scutari Press is a division of Scutari Projects Ltd, the publishing company
of the Royal College of Nursing.

First published 1995

British Library Cataloguing in Publication Data

Wright, Stephen G.
  Nursing Development Units
I. Title II. Salvage, Jane
610.73

  ISBN 1-873853-25-4

Typeset by CBS, Felixstowe, Suffolk
Printed by Bell and Bain Ltd, Glasgow

Contents

Contributors

Gillian Black BA, RN, DN, PGCEA
Independent Consultant in Primary Health Care Nursing

Rebecca Malby RGN, DipN, MA
Director of Nursing Practice, Institute of Nursing, University of
Leeds

Alan Pearson RN, RNT, MSc, PhD, FRCNA, FRCN
Professor of Nursing, University of New England, Australia

Jane Salvage RN, BA, MSc
Regional Adviser for Nursing and Midwifery, Regional Office for
Europe, World Health Organization

Barbara Vaughan RN, RNT, MSc
Director, Nursing Developments, King's Fund Centre for Health
Services Development

Stephen G Wright RN, RNT, DipN, DANS, MSc, FRCN, MBE
Director, The European Nursing Development Agency (TENDA)
and Visiting Professor of Nursing, University of Southampton

Preface

Nursing development units (NDUs) have existed by that name in the UK since the early 1980s. Many other nursing settings – wards, clinics, community teams – share their philosophy and aims, although they may not use the title. The work of the NDUs at Burford, Tameside and Oxford is already well known to British nurses, and from 1988 the movement was given further impetus through projects launched with the help of or supported by the King's Fund Centre Nursing Developments Programme. Contacts have been made and ideas exchanged with nurses working in similar ways in the USA and, increasingly, in other countries in Europe.

The publicity in the nursing press, at conferences and in the national media demonstrates the interest, enthusiasm and sometimes controversy generated by NDUs. We therefore thought it timely to produce a book that gives an update on progress so far: to explode some of the myths, reflect on the issues, celebrate the successes, explore the challenges and answer some of the questions frequently asked about NDUs. Thus, we shall explore some of the defining factors of NDUs, the historical backdrop, the achievements and problems and suggested future pathways. Our intention is to produce a guide of value to nurses actively involved in clinical practice development rather than to produce an academic study, although the contributors of course refer to theoretical work as well as to their own involvement with NDUs.

Two research studies – funded by the Department of Health, managed by the King's Fund Centre and undertaken by Mary Black and Janet Turner-Shaw – were published after this book was completed. Turner-Shaw studied the work of the four 'King's Fund pilot' NDUs (Brighton, Camberwell, Southport and West Dorset) between 1989 and 1992, while Black studied Tameside NDU in 1990–2, plus a retrospective evaluation). In addition, many NDUs are now publishing their own accounts in the professional press. All this work complements and deepens the insights recorded in this book.

The very fact of the contributors' direct involvement with NDUs meant that the gestation of the book was longer than intended, since busy lives leave little time for writing. Furthermore, both editors changed jobs in the course of the writing to posts that support nursing development but on a larger, European scale, giving a different perspective on the British NDU scene. We apologise to our patient publishers and to those long-suffering contributors who did meet their original deadlines.

So many people have contributed their ideas and energies to the NDU movement that it is impossible to acknowledge them all. First and foremost, nurses, midwives and health visitors in the units themselves shared their thoughts and experiences, especially those at Burford, Oxford, Tameside and the King's Fund NDUs at Brighton, Camberwell, Southport and West Dorset, while Linda Dineen, Brenda Hawkey and Eileen Hills contributed case studies. The Sainsbury Family Charitable Trusts, King Edward's Hospital Fund for London, the Department of Health, England, and individual health authorities gave generous funds to help launch the units. Robin Coates, Sue Coates, Hugh de Quetteville, Marie Manthey, Robert Maxwell and Barbara Stocking gave support and expertise. Patrick West, former editor at Scutari Press, persuaded the editors to embark on the book over a jolly good lunch at Heal's.

Finally, we dedicate this book to the memory of Bob Tiffany, our friend and colleague, whose inspired leadership over many years at the Royal Marsden Hospitals helped to put clinical practice development on the British nursing map.

Jane Salvage and Steve Wright

CHAPTER 1

Nursing Development Units in Context

Stephen G Wright

For many years little attention was paid to developing nursing practice. Changes and innovations had occurred, but these were often piecemeal and isolated. However, by the late 1970s a gathering momentum for change in nursing had begun in the UK, with some common themes emerging: new expectations of nurses and patients, expanding educational opportunities and a shift towards more patient-centred forms of practice.

These and other features made a force for change in nursing, so that by the late 1980s Salvage (1990) was able to describe the phenomenon as the 'New Nursing' – a wide-ranging movement with many elements focusing on the empowerment of nurses, the management of change and patient-centred care. Other evidence supports the view that a movement for change was well under way. Reports from the Audit Commission (1991), York University (Carr-Hill et al 1992) and the North–Western Regional Health Authority (1992), while indicating that qualified nurses are cost-effective, also revealed the extent to which nurses were changing their practices. In the early 1980s about 75 per cent of all nursing care in hospitals, and to some extent in the community, was delivered by task allocation. Already dismissed by Briggs (1972) as 'the production-line concept of care', task allocation had come to dominate nursing. Care, divided into a number of procedures linked to a medical diagnosis, was fragmented among a number of nurses.

Patients and nurses found this fundamentally unsatisfactory. The desire to deliver more holistic care led nurses to re-examine the way their work was organised. Within ten years a massive shift had taken place, moving nurses away from task-based methods of work to more patient-focused ones. By the late 1980s task allocation as the dominant mode had collapsed and over 80 per cent of nurses

1

were using work methods designed to facilitate patient-centred care, such as team nursing, patient allocation, case management and primary nursing.

Changing the way nurses organise their practice is not a guarantee of patient-centred care. It is also necessary to examine nurses' values and beliefs about themselves and their patients. An organisational method gives nurses the opportunity to shift the focus of their attention, but does not guarantee that they will behave differently. Thus, in parallel with a reorganisation of practice, there has been a re-examination of the philosophies and values about nurses and nursing that underpin the way each nurse works.

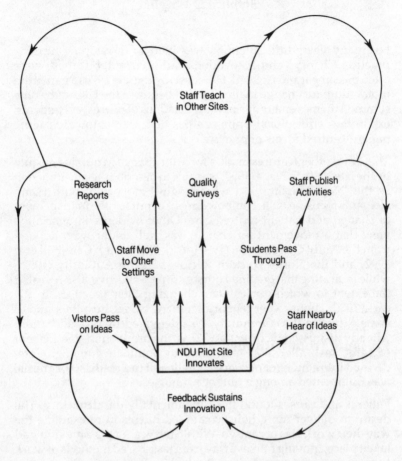

Figure 1.1 Dissemination – NDUs influence other settings

Nursing development units both have been a response to this pursuit of change and have given it further stimulus. They contributed significantly to the dissemination of knowledge about patient-centred practice and innovation in care. Clearly, they were not the only ones doing so, but a glance through the nursing literature or the conference and workshop programmes of the mid- to late 1980s suggests that NDUs were making a significant contribution to change in nursing and continue to do so. Yet nursing has not moved logically from one innovation to the next. History tends to be viewed as a series of milestone events which determine the future or in terms of great people striving to succeed against overwhelming odds. Many nursing histories see nursing as an almost self-congratulatory progress 'out of the dark ages, to the present, modern times' (Davies 1980). In reality change is often messy and unpredictable and, as in the case of NDUs, the boundaries between cause and effect are blurred.

The development of nursing practice is by no means exclusive to NDUs. In an enormous range of settings, nurses are making innovations in practice and developing new roles, such as clinical nurse specialists, nurse practitioners and community psychiatric nurses. Studies and research projects have multiplied and individual nurses, specialised units, progressive educational centres and professional bodies have all contributed to the crucible of change. Strategy documents setting out a vision and goals for nursing have emerged from a variety of sources. But however described or focused, all these strategies share a common vision for nursing, based on patient-centred approaches, the desire to improve the quality of care, the willingness to experiment, professional autonomy and accountability and the expansion and extension of nursing knowledge, roles and practices. In NDUs, all these elements are fused into a common commitment to pursue a vision of nursing and to undertake the changes necessary to reach that vision.

Pressure from without

Changes within nursing have also been accelerated by external events. The 1980s saw a series of major reorganisations of the National Health Service and the expansion of the independent sector. The most recent NHS reforms have yet to be fully realised, but NHS trusts are now the norm and the spread of clinical directorates has increased the demand for effective nurse leaders. The first *Patient's Charter* was published in the 1991 (DoH 1991), followed by the Government White Paper, *The Health of the Nation*

(DoH 1992). Both have major implications for nursing roles and practices. Major input is needed from nurses to act as patient advocates, information-givers and partners in care.

Nurses remain the largest single group of employees in health care, consuming up to half its resources in their salaries alone. They are present in almost every health care setting and have considerable influence on the way resources are used. A growing awareness of these factors has led government and managers to focus much more sharply on nurses and what they do, with a variable response. Nurses have often reacted with suspicion – particularly when they perceive that a re-examination of their roles is motivated by the desire to cut costs rather than to improve the quality of patient care. There has also been much support for nursing practice innovation, reinforced by a growing body of evidence that nurses who are supported in their development, provided with good leadership and a responsive management climate and given opportunities to practise in patient-centred ways are cost-effective (Price Waterhouse 1988, Audit Commission 1991, Buchan and Ball 1991, Carr-Hill et al 1992). To some extent this has overturned the myth that cheaper pairs of hands are all that is needed to produce cost-effective health care. When adequately supported, the qualified nurse is able to make decisions, innovate and deliver care efficiently and effectively.

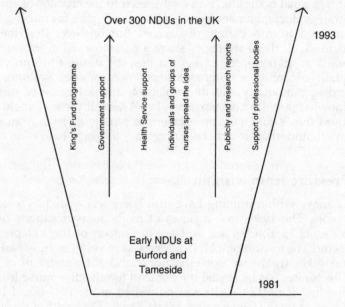

Figure 1.2 NDUs increase in number

A growing awareness of all these factors, some astute lobbying by nurse leaders and professional bodies and a growing body of evidence eventually led to overt support for nursing developments during the 1980s. The then Secretary of State for Health, William Waldegrave, and the chief executive of the National Health Service, Duncan Nichol, actively encouraged the setting up of more NDUs, with a grant of £3.5 million announced in 1991, to be managed by the King's Fund Centre.

The Patient's Charter (DoH 1991) reinforced the concept of the 'named nurse', in the first major public policy statement that each patient should have his or her own named nurse, midwife or health visitor responsible for his or her care. The significance of this should not be underestimated, for this document is in the public domain and will influence people's expectations of their entitlements to health care. It also represents acceptance of a value which underlay all the early NDUs and their nursing practice initiatives. An issue which had previously seemed controversial had now moved into the mainstream, become accepted and was high on the political agenda.

Meanwhile, support for other nursing practice initiatives has continued in a variety of ways. These include national and local award schemes, such as the Yorkshire Regional Health Authority's small grants and practice development projects.

Valuing nursing, valuing nurses

Within this maelstrom of change other factors have also been at work. Nursing does not exist in isolation, but mirrors the values and beliefs of the wider society. However, there is one way in which nursing is not representative of society: in terms of numbers it is heavily skewed as an occupation employing women (90 per cent). Thus any social changes that re-evaluate the role of women and women's work eventually spill over into nursing. The future of nursing and other caring professions in which women predominate is intimately bound to the future of women and to any re-evaluation of the nature and significance of caring. The traditional model dismisses caring as 'just women's work', conforming to the public stereotype of 'a girl who bathes people and gives out bedpans' (Hector 1973). The link between the 'girl' and what is seen as a menial task is significant, for the relationship between nurses and doctors is still characterised by a dominance–subservience, master–servant model. Doctoring was traditionally dominated by men and nursing by women, in terms of numbers. In addition, the male view of the world and of illness and health care has predominated, reinforced by class and racial divisions, doctors being drawn predominately from white upper-middle-class backgrounds. Nursing came to be seen as an adjunct to medicine, keeping the patient clean and fed while the doctor did the important work of effecting a cure through a seemingly complex decision-making and technological process regarded as beyond the grasp of most women.

The arrival of women in medicine, of men in nursing, the challenging of media stereotypes of nursing, and so on – all have questioned the status quo and are continuing to do so (Stein 1990). The issue concerns not only the numbers of one sex in the profession, but also the value that is attached to what nurses do. Within nursing there has been a growing recognition that nursing is more than a medical add-on; it has a healing and therapeutic function in its own right. Nurses may be involved in carrying out medical regimens, but they are also concerned with caring. Indeed, while caring is not exclusive to nursing, nursing is the only discipline that makes caring its *raison d'être*.

Traditionally this 'caring' has been subsumed within the medical model. Thus hi-tech aspects of care acquired more status and were seen as more demanding and complex. This view is shared by many nurses and has spilled over into the wider community. Many influential managers and health policy-makers see health care in this light. Nurses may be lured by the 'narcissistic mirror offered by medicine' (Oakley 1984), producing a hierarchy of nursing in which those elements associated with cure and technical intervention receive the greatest attention, resources, acclaim and status, while other elements – the expressive and comforting ones, described by Benner (1984) as 'presencing' – may be dismissed as simple and menial.

NDUs have been in the vanguard of challenging these views. They are a product of a trend towards greater equality in nursing and a re-examination of its roles and nature, and a further stimulus to both. Thus NDUs commonly adopt and practise equal opportunities policies and accept that all dimensions of nursing are intricate and complex. They have played a significant role in developing the idea of nursing as a therapy. The traditional view of the nature of nursing is therefore being challenged from within nursing and to some extent from outside too. Part of the strategy for developing nursing practice is to accept the therapeutic value of nursing and to develop practices and research that can illuminate this. Evaluating practice also forms a crucial element of NDU work, which will contribute significantly to determining the success of this movement. There is also considerable work to be done – to which NDUs can contribute – in stimulating this reappraisal of the value of nursing among those who are not nurses, those who control health care organisations and society's resources.

Conclusion

The picture of recent nursing development is complex. NDUs form one significant part of this puzzle. They may be seen as a response to demands from within and outside nursing for changes in nursing practice. They are also making their contributions to the debate and the change in various ways – developing clinical leadership and promoting equal opportunities, setting a clear vision for nursing and examining and expanding its role, developing strategies for change, evaluating practice and promoting its value. They provide a melting pot for change whose influence will spread far beyond the local unit.

Nursing and the health care system have recently experienced an accelerating pace of change, creating an environment that is ripe for nurses to respond to and capitalise on these changes. Through the NDU movement, nurses can contribute to making clear the value of nursing – a crucial role in the new world of health care where market forces will be increasingly important. NDUs will help to empower nurses with the knowledge and skills they need, not only to deliver cost-effective, high quality care, but also to meet the challenge of the political and social agenda and argue successfully for the support and expansion of the profession.

The focus of NDUs is the recognition that to develop nursing, it is also necessary to develop nurses. Nurses constitute the greatest number of health care workers; therefore, any improvements they may bring can have a major impact on health care overall, probably more than introducing change in any other single discipline.

An NDU demonstrates that caring need not cost more and indeed, by recruiting and retaining well-motivated and skilled staff, it can contain costs far better than settings that do not meet the standards of the NDU. The aspirations and aims of NDUs seem to have many common elements. What drives them above all is a commitment to changing nursing practice and a shared vision of the future – a better future for both patients and nurses. NDUs do not claim to be centres of excellence, but they do aspire to it.

The potential benefits to patients and nurses are not without problems. Some managers, doctors and others may find it difficult to cope with more assertive, knowledgeable and empowered nurses. They may make greater demands for knowledge, education and the freedom to practise. Many nurses may respond to the NDU with praise, support and a willingness to learn from it, but others may display jealousy, hostility, a refusal to accept its ideas – the common responses when we fear change or find it difficult to acknowledge the work of leaders and pioneers. Organisational support, too, can have its problems. For example, the NHS Management Executive Objectives (1993) state that 'the spread of Nursing Development Units and the good practice they foster, should be encouraged'. Thus, good intentions of organisational support may lead to increased pressure on nurses to create NDUs by management, 'top-down' edict, rather than allow gradual, 'bottom-up' growth from the clinical level. Subsequent chapters will explore in more detail the defining characteristics of NDUs, how to go about setting one up and how to manage change.

Furthermore, developing nurses has implications beyond the NDU site. There is a knock-on effect outside the profession. Empowered and developed nurses may question their personal and domestic ties and the social status quo. NDUs can also contribute to the development of the service as a whole and to other disciplines. When nurses are clear about their own value and vision, they are in a better position to work collaboratively.

NDUs are more than a fixed ward, department or locality – these serve only to provide the clinical focus for its activities. The NDU is the people who work in it, what they do, how they relate to each other and their clients and how they change themselves and their practices.

Some NDUs are more mature than others and not all will meet the criteria listed in subsequent chapters. Many NDUs will be at different stages of development, but they share a commitment to pursue common goals. It is important to remember that the NDU concept is not a nursing *developed* unit but a nursing *development* unit. The latter relates to the nature of the NDU as an evolving entity, not fixed and having achieved in full all its goals as the former would imply.

NDUs are one means among many by which change can be wrought in nursing practice. There are other options which may be more appropriate in different settings. They are not panaceas; they will not cure nursing's ills overnight. However, they do have a crucial role to play in liberating nursing to develop creative, compassionate caring, to think about, explore, value and enjoy nursing.

In the future, when all nurses practise excellent, thoughtful, creative, high quality nursing – and are supported in all ways to do so – NDUs may become redundant, for then every setting will accept that change is a way of life and the support of nurses to achieve perfection will have been accomplished. Even so, there will probably always be a need for centres of clinical nursing to research and explore its boundaries. Meanwhile, NDUs have a role to play. They may not yet embody perfection in nursing, but they do aim for it and offer hope and encouragement to others to do likewise.

References

Audit Commission (1991) *The Virtue of Patients.* London: Audit Commission.
Benner P (1984) *From Novice to Expert.* New York: Addison-Wesley.
Briggs A (Chair) (1972) *Report of the Committee on Nursing.* London: HMSO.
Buchan J and Ball J (1991) *Caring Costs.* IMS Report No. 128. University of Sussex: Institute of Manpower Studies.
Carr-Hill R, Dixon P, Gibbs I, Griffiths M, Higgins M, McCaughan D and Wright K (1992) *Skill Mix and the Effectiveness of Care.* University of York: Centre for Health Economics.
Davies C (1980) *Rewriting Nursing History.* London: Croom Helm.
Department of Health (1991) *The Patient's Charter.* London: HMSO.
Department of Health (1992) *The Health of the Nation.* London: HMSO.
Hector W (1973) *The Work of Mrs Bedford Fenwick and the Rise of Professional Nursing.* London: Royal College of Nursing.
NHSME (1993) *Objectives 1993–1994.* Leeds: National Health Service Management Executive.
North Western Regional Health Authority (1992) *Ward Nursing Quality and Grade Mix.* Manchester: NWRHA.
Oakley A (1984) The importance of being a nurse. *Nursing Times* **80**(50): 24–27.
Price Waterhouse (1988) *Recruitment and Retention of Nurses* (Report commissioned by the Department of Health). London: Price Waterhouse.
Salvage J (1990) The theory and practice of the 'New Nursing'. *Nursing Times* **86**(4): 42–45.
Stein L I (1990) The doctor–nurse game revisited. *The New England Journal of Medicine* **322**(8): 546–549.

CHAPTER 2

Developing Nursing – creativity and change

Stephen G Wright

In Chapter 1 it was suggested that the pace of change in nursing had accelerated remarkably since the early 1980s. In addition, many of the health service organisations in which nurses work have undergone radical reformation.

Considerable advance seems to have taken place in the way nurses organise their work. The shift from task-focused to patient-centred care during the 1980s was dramatic and appears to be continuing. It needs to be remembered, however, that not all sectors of nursing have changed at the same pace. Indeed, some would argue that they had no need to change the way they delivered care because they already worked in patient-centred ways. This seems to apply particularly to health visitors and most community nurses, for example.

Even so, this leaves little room for complacency. First, because care is organised in patient-centred ways, this is no guarantee the care will *de facto* be more personal. The chosen organisational method, such as team nursing or primary nursing, is clearly a critical factor, which puts the nurse in a position to treat the patient as an individual, to assess, plan, give and evaluate care more personally and to accept authority and accountability for practice. But there are other factors at work too. Martin's (1984) research suggests that nurses' ability to deliver care that is tailored to individual needs is also affected by:

- The presence of an effective nurse leader at the clinical level
- Positive managerial support
- Involvement of clinical staff in organisational decision-making
- Opportunities for continued professional development
- The resources available and the suitability of the environment

in which care takes place
* The values which they themselves hold about their client group, nursing and nurses

In other words, it seems that reorganising patient care through patient-centred methods will not necessarily make care more personal. Nurses need an organisational culture and environment that enables and supports them as individuals in the performance of their work. They also need to have a clear vision of nursing and health care and what their part in it is. Values drive practice. What nurses believe about themselves and their clients will ultimately affect the way they work.

Nursing is a practice discipline; therefore there are major implications for the ideas and beliefs that nurses have about nursing. If nursing were purely theoretical, then the effect of nurses' values and beliefs might be minimal. Because nursing requires nurses to act on their beliefs, what they believe about themselves and their practice directly affects the lives of their patients.

This supports Manthey's (1980) view that systems such as primary nursing are not just methods of organising care, but are also philosophies of care. Consider the hypothetical example of a nurse working in a care of the elderly unit, but who dislikes elderly people and has difficulty seeing them as individuals. She has little belief that they still have scope for growth and development and takes the pessimistic view that they are at the end of their lives and have little need of personal attention or nursing intervention. No matter what organisational method of patient-centred care is in place, a nurse such as this is unlikely to treat her patients as individuals, simply because she does not believe in them or the part she might play in therapeutic interventions with them.

Such negative values about particular patient groups lead some nurses to practise depersonalised care. It develops in some instances into rigid, institutionalised approaches to care (Martin 1984, Ashworth Hospital Inquiry 1992) even, in the extreme, to downright cruelty. Nurses in Nazi Germany participated in the extermination programmes for the mentally ill, the mentally handicapped and the chronically sick (Lifton 1986, Müller-Hill 1988).

Fortunately, such extremes are relatively rare occurrences; more often the failings form part of a daily, low-level inattentiveness to the patient as an individual. This forms the backcloth of regular complaints to health organisations (Health Service Ombudsman

1986–91). Patients seem to complain not so much about major abuses of care, but about feeling ignored or overlooked as individuals. It may be the nurse on the busy surgical ward, thinking about patients in the context of the medical model, who tends to treat one appendicectomy just like the next. It may be the nurse in the patient's home who rushes the patient through her bath in order to get the work done. Whatever the setting, the underlying cause is often the same – a lack of awareness on the part of nurses about their values and how these are transmitted to their patients and clients.

Some of the literature cited above and in Chapter 1 suggests that nurses have been advancing their practice along the continuum from institutionalised to individualised approaches to care. The former is dominated by rigid routines, an absence of personally planned care and the treatment of patients according to illness categories and diagnosis. There is also a trend towards a hierarchical organisation of care, which restricts an individual nurse's contact, personal relationship and autonomy with individual patients.

The latter suggests a breakdown of rigid routines, a much more flexible system of organisation and patient/client involvement in care. Care is planned and organised to meet individual needs and authority is devolved to individual nurses to take responsibility for their own caseload of patients.

Nursing practice in recent years seems to have been moving more towards this individualised model of care. In so doing nurses not only change their practice, but also re-examine themselves. Once on this path nurses appear to enter what might be described as 'advanced' practice. They begin to learn and practise nursing as a therapeutic act (McMahon and Pearson 1991). The evidence from settings such as NDUs suggests that a veritable explosion of innovation takes place once values and practices begin to be questioned. Having changed some things, nurses appear to feel liberated and empowered to change even more. They experiment with self-medication schemes, give patients access to nursing information, begin to apply complementary therapies, set standards, assess quality of care, and so on. The boundaries of nursing knowledge and practice are rolled back as change is implemented and accelerates.

It has already been suggested that institutionalised and task-based methods of organising care are satisfying to neither nurses nor patients. Advanced practice moves away from this territory and has incorporated the antithesis of task-based methods into its everyday work. Benner (1984) characterises this as possessing:

- The recognition and application of nursing as a therapeutic act
- Treatment and regard for the patient as an individual
- Nurses using highly developed technical and interpersonal skills (the expressive and the instrumental) to work with the patient in partnership
- High levels of teaching, counselling, supporting and involvement of the patient/others in care
- The ability of nurses to 'be with' patients and 'bear witness' ('presencing'), so that patients see their nurse as an ally in their health care. Such an approach is of itself healing to patients

Campbell (1984) describes such a highly developed form of practice as 'moderated love'; Peplau (1952) calls it 'professional friendship'. The nurse works with such empathy and skill that problem-solving and helping to care are transcended to the point that the nature of the helping relationship between nurse and patient becomes a therapeutic act in itself (McMahon and Pearson 1991).

It seems logical to assume that this helping relationship, which will vary in degree with each individual patient's needs and wishes, is what patients would wish for. Most nurses would expect it for themselves if they were patients. NDUs are committed to the development of therapeutic nursing, which is by its very nature an 'advance' on the depersonalised, institutional mould. In doing so, NDUs not only focus on changing particular modes or practice, but also conduct a gradual reappraisal of nursing values. For, as has already been suggested, the two are intimately linked.

Changing nursing practice

The use of the word 'development' in NDUs is itself indicative of change. It is an explicit term, which indicates that nursing is being questioned and sometimes being tried, tested and evaluated. Challenging nursing practices and developing an individualised philosophy of nursing in each nurse suggests that change, to a greater or lesser extent, is under way. If nurses have moved away significantly from task-centred to patient-centred methods of care, then, somewhere along the line, change has occurred. If NDUs have done this and more, then once again change is under way.

The way change is managed has great significance in relation to the success, or failure, of the outcome. Traditionally, change in nursing has often been quite haphazard, relying on the enthusiasm of groups of staff in small, localised settings, or the power of authority, or the energy and input of a new innovative nurse leader in place. There is a growing body of evidence to suggest that such approaches, in the long term, are ineffective. NDUs recognise that changing practices and attitudes requires a comprehensive, long-term change strategy. A number of models are available and are discussed at length elsewhere (Ottoway 1980, Turrill 1985, Wright 1989, Kitson et al 1990, Pearson 1992). Kitson (1990), for example, recognises that the process of standard-setting may stimulate nurses into changing their practice. Wright (1989) and Pearson (1992) advocate a planned approach to change, incorporating many elements. It is beyond the scope of this text to deal with change theory and its application in detail. However, a number of key points can be summarised which are commonly incorporated into the work of NDUs.

Any proposed changes are planned

Planning change will not avoid all the pitfalls – the change process is far too volatile for that. However, it will help to mitigate difficulties, give structure, meaning and direction to what is happening and provide a means of evaluating what is taking place.

In many respects, the cycle is not unlike that of the nursing process:

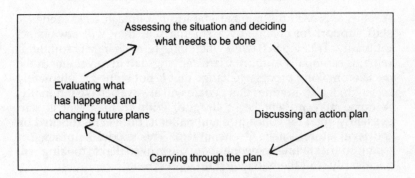

Figure 2.1 The cycle of change

At the same time it is recognised that the change process is rarely as linear as this. Indeed, one of the hallmarks of those who succeed is their ability to respond flexibly to problems as they arise, to think and act creatively and to modify plans in the light of changing circumstances. Lewin (1958) describes how the team can be brought together, to discuss new ideas to help 'unfreeze' established thinking and ways of doing things. 'Movement' then takes place in people's thinking and behaviour, until they 'refreeze' into the new style or way of thinking/behaving. Ottoway (1980) identifies the key role of the lead change agent who helps guide and facilitate the changes, while recognising that all, in participating in the change process, are agents of change themselves. Turrill (1985) describes how plans of change can 'map the environment' and how nurses can tap into the organisation to gain support and resources. All these elements in change have had their work developed and applied successfully by Wright (1989) and Pearson (1992). A common thread running through all these texts is the importance of the role of the clinical leader/change agent and the engagement of the whole team in the process of change.

The changes are 'bottom-up'

Organisations and individuals often seek to implement change by the use of authority, to force its adoption. This 'power-coercive' method may succeed in producing some change in the short term, but ultimately it fails. Staff may modify their behaviour to comply with the manager's wishes, but they may ultimately reject and subvert it because they do not share in it – they do not 'own' it.

Another approach, the 'rational–empirical' approach, seeks to engage staff support for change by assuming that they will always act rationally. This too is flawed when long-term change is sought. It remains essentially authoritarian, denying staff involvement in the decision-making process. (Change that is not owned is ultimately rejected.) It also assumes that people will always behave rationally. A nurse may present her colleagues with an idea that is self-evidently good for colleagues and patients, but yet be shocked by the level of resistance it encounters. This model assumes, for example, that telling someone about the proven ills of smoking will necessarily lead them to give it up forever!

NDUs, while reaffirming that many change strategies need to be used to manage the highly unpredictable course of change, tend to espouse a bottom-up method (the 'normative–re-educative') which engages all the staff in the process of change and seeks their cooperation and commitment in the long term, so that they feel they 'own' what is happening.

The creation of the NDU itself needs to be 'bottom-up', not just the changes that it undertakes. It is necessary for nurses first to be clear what an NDU is, how it can help them and what they hope to achieve by it. Setting up an NDU is itself a process of change which needs careful planning to minimise conflicts and misunderstanding. To help think through some of these issues, my colleagues at TENDA produced some guidance steps:

Setting up an NDU – Minimising the Pain of the Process

1. Build knowledge on the subject among your colleagues and yourself first. Attend workshops on the subject, read the relevant literature, visit an NDU, seek advice from people experienced in the field, e.g. clinical leaders in NDUs or King's Fund Network. Lobby. Discuss. Debate.

2. Spend time sharing ideas at team meetings and building up a consensus of what an NDU is. Ask yourself, and answer, the following questions:
   (a) What is an NDU – are we clear about it?
   (b) Why do we want it?
   (c) How will it help us?
   (d) What will it do to improve patient care/outcomes?
   (e) What alternatives for innovation can we use and would any of these be better than an NDU to achieve our goals?
   (f) Who will be the clinical leader?
   (g) What do we expect the NDU to do? (Identify at least ten things.)

3. If you're sure an NDU is the right way forward for you, then set up a small coordination team to produce an action plan.

4. Once an action plan has been agreed, produce clear, written proposals about the NDU – what it will be/do; results expected; projects planned; education links; evaluation plans, etc. (See the text listing the defining characteristics of the NDU.)

5. Keep the dialogue going with team members, educators and managers so that everyone is up-to-date on the direction.

6. Agree proposals with the team/the organisation.

7. Create an advisory board to guide (but not manage) the NDU. Involve, especially, clinicians and others whose support is needed – doctors, chief executives, etc. Let someone who also supports the NDU and who has influence within the organisation chair this committee.

8. Allow time for all this process to be pursued – perhaps 12–18 months.

Continues

---

9. Consider applying for grants, special funds, etc., if this is necessary to boost resources for research and projects, for example.
10. Clarify and review the philosophy, objectives/goals of the NDU. Set up a work plan detailing objectives, completion dates, strategies, lead persons and so on. Review this at every coordination meeting of the team.
11. Consider including a team-building strategy before and after the NDU is under way.
12. Make sure that everyone who wishes to do so has a role to play – make the contribution explicit in your work plan. Try to ensure that everyone is included.

Such a bottom-up approach appears to be the most effective way of producing long-term, permanent and meaningful change in nursing. It is a common feature of all NDUs that a collective and collaborative approach to change is under way. Managers, educators and others also have a role to play in facilitating and enabling the change to take place, but they cannot control it. The on-site clinical team, acting collectively and guided by the clinical leader/change agent and supported by managers and educators, emerges as a powerful force for change in nursing.

Change is supported by planned programmes of personal and professional development

NDUs are committed to develop nursing. To do so they must also develop nurses. This includes not only increasing nurses' skill and knowledge in nursing practice, but also developing the nurse as a person. Plans for staff development include teaching methods which take account of personal growth and awareness, assertiveness, decision-making and change management.

A variety of organisational means to develop staff in this way is available. Well-known NDUs at Tameside and Burford, for example, made use of counsellors, psychotherapists, reflective practice, clinical supervision, role-modelling and drama techniques to raise staff awareness of themselves and their part in nursing. Creative and questioning practice demands the production of creative and questioning practitioners. Formal courses, conferences and workshops have a part to play, but developing the personal skills and attributes of the nurse requires more tailor-made and personal approaches. It needs to be remembered that what is being challenged is not just the status quo of nursing practice, but the values and attitudes of nurses themselves.

Such changes cannot be brought about in 'quick-fix' class-room lectures. Highly skilled facilitators and time set aside for development are needed to help nurses reappraise themselves and their roles. Some nurses can arrive at such a level of expertise by dint of their own experience and abilities to reflect on their practice. For others, much more structured and deliberate plans need to be brought into play. NDUs tap into a whole range of options to help nurses change not just their practices, but themselves.

Once the process of change is under way in NDUs, it is often characterised by its breadth and scope. It is also frequently incremental, as one change stimulates many others. The following summary illustrates this point with reference to the original Tameside NDU. However, a similar pattern might be found in any of the current NDUs. A number of factors were identified as essential characteristics of the NDU. These are listed below, along with brief details of the events that took place in the Tameside NDU.

The NDU focuses on:

1. The concept of *nursing as a therapy*. It seeks to explore its boundaries.

   Recognised in the original work on the philosophy of nursing by the staff. Many subsequent projects (e.g. changing the management climate, applying primary nursing, piloting nursing beds, etc.). Sought to explore the organisation of care to facilitate the application of nursing as a therapy. Skill mix changed to increase number of qualified staff.

2. Developing the *autonomy* of nurses and the autonomy of the NDU itself to pursue its goals.

   The NDU was a self-managed unit. Nursing roles were defined. The dependent–interdependent–dependent relationship to medicine clarified. Staff development work sought to reinforce this. Nursing projects were set up and led by nurses.

3. A *clinical base* where nurses and patients are working together in a defined setting, with the work of the NDU being led by the nursing team.

   Based in a clinical setting (the care of older people with acute health problems). The NDU was created and led by clinical nurses.

4. A manageable *size* for the NDU – beginning small on one ward, but later pursuing agreed expansion.

   Began on one ward, but expanded over ten years, with agreement of others, to include nine wards and a day hospital. Other nearby units affiliated to it, contributed to knowledge and spread of NDUs nationwide.

5. Using a *change* strategy, involving a bottom-up approach, with team members' responsibilities clearly defined and based on a work plan of aims and objectives.

   Change agents appointed and a 'bottom-up' change strategy used (based on the work of Ottoway, Lewin and Turrill). Clinical staff at ward level defined and controlled the changes. Managers and educators acted as facilitators. Programme of changes documented. Changes continued, new ideas constantly being introduced. The NDU itself changed in nature, structure and goals.

6. Developing a *nursing culture* of shared philosophy, team spirit, goals, values, commitment to change and passion and excitement for nursing.

   Nursing culture emerged which broke away from the old, ritualised, institutionalised mould, generating commitment to change and new interests in nursing.

7. Agreeing, documenting and reviewing its *philosophy*.

   Philosophy documented and reviewed every two years. Used to underpin work on standards, the nursing model, objectives for change, etc. Used in staff recruitment, team-building. Available to public.

8. Developing its own *nursing model*.

   Developed and documented over a four-year period.

9. *Exploration* of nursing through a multiplicity of projects and research.

   Multiplicity of projects pursued with staff involved at all levels, e.g. primary nursing, self-medication, out-of-uniform trials, pet therapy, complementary therapies, standard-setting, patient access to nursing records, designing patient information books, changing ward routines, patient teaching plans, care planning system, etc. Some staff led projects, others supported them. Funding pursued to support some projects. Planning and evaluation carried out.

10. *New roles* for nurses and developing nursing-led services.

New roles for nursing explored – primary nursing, continence adviser, clinical specialists, consultant nurse, ethnic needs worker, reminiscence therapist, etc. Practices developed to include some work previously undertaken by doctors, appropriate roles of support workers identified (e.g. ward clerks), expansion of nursing role. Skill mix changed to increase proportions of qualified staff.

11. *Research* application – carrying out studies, reviewing findings and applying research to practice.

Variety of projects pursued, from small-scale ones to others undertaken as part of course fulfilment – MSc and PhD theses. Staff attended ENB research courses. Clinical specialists and consultant had research advisory roles. Research forum formed. Journals purchased. Research fundings applied.

12. Defining *clinical leaders* and exploring, clarifying and developing their roles.

Clinical leader appointed (initially jointly appointed nurse-tutor and charge nurse, later to become consultant nurse). Each ward identified its own clinical leader with further development. Resources controlled by NDU team. Development plans included for other team members.

13. *Empowerment* of patients through information sharing and many strategies/projects developed with this goal in mind.

Information sharing policy developed, including access to nursing records, standard of care, information centres, information books, etc. Patient committees formed. Advice of external agents sought (e.g. Age Concern).

14. *Partnership* in care with multidisciplinary team, within the nursing team as well as between patients, nurses and other carers.

Primary nurses work as partners with patients. Code of behaviour agreed among team and documented. Multidisciplinary team involved in many aspects of the NDU's activities, including social occasions, shared learning opportunities, joint project work, etc.

15. *Patient-centred care* by choosing the best methods of organising care, challenging routines and rituals and emphasising creativity and change.

Total realignment of clinical activity took place to break the institutional mould and produced a more patient-centred climate. Modification to environment (improvements to buildings, decor, furniture, etc.) made. Primary nursing, self-medication schemes, etc. underway.

16. The *involvement* of other carers such as collaborative projects with the multidisciplinary team, identifying shared learning opportunities and developing strategies to involve relatives and friends.

Collaborative work undertaken in many areas. Age Concern representatives invited to form advocacy scheme. Guidelines for relatives' participation in care agreed. Relative/patient teaching plans developed. Ward routines reorganised to permit maximum participation (e.g. lifting of rigid visiting times).

17. *Equality* in caring, emphasising care that is non-discriminating and ensuring equal opportunities policy for staff.

Included in ward philosophy and monitored through evaluation process. Ethnic specialist appointed. Authority equal opportunities regulations applied and monitored.

18. *Organisational support* with explicit commitment at managerial level, agreeing NDU activities with managers and seeking guidance and support through an advisory board.

Agreed, in writing, after negotiation at all levels. One manager had specific remit to support the NDU. NDU trustees and advisory board created. The clinical leader was a member of this board.

19. *Financial resources*: the NDU works with defined and agreed resources, with any additional monies for specific NDU projects controlled by the NDU. The NDU actively income-generating to support projects (e.g. by applying for research grants).

Budget allocation defined. Ward budgets created. Trust funds set up. Income generation plan put into action (e.g. study days, visitors' fees, sale of information packs and other items, consultancy fees charged, etc.).

20. *Staff development* with an agreed strategy and a variety of options available. It is open to all staff and has links with several post-graduate educational settings.

Wide-ranging strategy agreed. Staff ordered off-site courses and conferences, from short seminars to full-time degree programmes. Courses designed for all grades of staff from nursing auxiliaries to qualified staff. Special courses for clinical leaders led by psychotherapist, including residential weekend. Therapists also undertook personal growth and awareness courses for other staff.

On-site library developed. Open learning packages provided. Staff teaching and careers counselling roles identified (e.g. consultant nurse and clinical specialists). Many on-site workshops and study programmes devised. Clinical supervision and reflective practice introduced. Support derived from links with a university department of nursing and the local college of nursing, technical college and polytechnic. International exchange schemes developed.

21. *Dissemination* using a variety of methods of outreach work, with a commitment to share knowledge and publication of results.

    Enormous amount of publicity generated (over 500 publications and press reports in ten years). Radio and TV contributions. Staff delivered many conference papers, led workshops, etc. NDU visitors' days set up. Information packs prepared. Longer placement offered to students, visitors, etc. Staff networked with others in the speciality, lobbied MPs, attended local support groups, and so on. Many staff active in professional organisations (e.g. RCN).

22. *Evaluation* using a multifaceted approach built into all projects. This includes standard-setting and monitoring, documenting the NDU's history, gathering baseline data and later making comparisons, including patient, staff, etc. responses in the quality assurance strategy.

    NDU history evaluated by independent researcher. Nursing standards set. Quality assurance strategy developed. Quality assurance nurse appointed. All projects evaluated. Questionnaires for patients, staff, visitors and interview schedules devised. Baseline data compiled and compared annually (bed occupancy, pressure sore rates, incontinence levels, death rates, readmission rates, patient satisfaction comments, patient complaints, staff leavers surveys, etc.). Results published. Annual report produced.

Questioning and understanding the nature of nursing and nurses, planning and implementing change are all integral to the NDU movement. The implications, however, go far beyond mere changes in practice in the local setting. Changing nursing practice involves, to a greater or lesser extent, changing the nurse. The nurse is not just an isolated role which is stepped into as easily as a uniform. Helping nurses to change their values and practice must also set in train changes in themselves as persons. The assertive, knowledgeable, questioning and creative nurse is in a far better position to contribute to changes in nursing in the NDU. Inevitably, however, such changes spill over into their personal and social lives.

In becoming aware of themselves as nurses and as people, some may find themselves questioning not just their professional but also their personal lives. They may seek to effect changes in the wider society, becoming more politically active, in challenging established norms in the wider organisation in which they work. Halmos (1978) has noted how personal, professional and political change agent roles tend to overlap. The question arises, of course, as to how far the 'New Nursing' (Salvage 1990) will also produce the 'new nurse'.

Discussion about developing and empowering nurses usually receives positive acclaim, but such nurses will not be pillars of the establishment. They will question the status quo. They will want to change things. It may be wondered how far support for nursing developments extends when the 'new nurses' challenge the managers' decisions, demand resources, use their initiative! It remains to be seen how far support for the empowerment of nurses is a reality rather than mere lip-service.

There are over half a million working nurses in the UK. If the NDU and 'New Nursing' movement continues to gather momentum, it does not take too great a leap of the imagination to foresee the implications. Half a million empowered, assertive, creative, effective change agents (most of whom will be women) represent an immense force for change, not just in nursing or health care, but in society as a whole.

In the end, it is probably too late to stop the changes in nursing and nurses that are already under way. Time alone will tell how far the NDU movement, and its offspring and those it influences, will influence the world about them. One thing is certain – there is no going back.

References

Ashworth Hospital Inquiry (1992) *Report of the Committee of Inquiry into Complaints about Ashworth Hospital.* (Chair, Sir Louis Blom-Cooper QC). London: HMSO.

Benner P (1984) *From Novice to Expert.* New York: Addison-Wesley.

Campbell A V (1984) *Moderated Love.* London: SPCK.

Halmos P (1978) *The Personal and the Political: Social Work and Political Action.* London: Century-Hutchinson.

Health Service Ombudsman (1986–91) *Reports of the Health Service Parliamentary Liaison Officer* (Ombudsman). London: Department of Health.

Kitson A L, Hyndman S J, Harvey G and Yerrell P H (1990) *Quality Patient*

Care: The Dynamic Standard Setting System. London: Scutari Press.
Lewin K (1958) The Group's Reason and Social Change. In E MacCoby (Ed.) *Readings in Social Psychology.* London: Holt, Rinehart and Winston.
Lifton R J (1986) *The Nazi Doctors.* London: Macmillan.
McMahon R and Pearson A (1991) *Nursing as Therapy.* London: Chapman & Hall.
Manthey M (1980) *The Practice of Primary Nursing.* Oxford: Blackwell.
Martin J P (1984) *Hospitals in Trouble.* Oxford: Blackwell.
Müller-Hill B (1988) *Murderous Science.* Oxford: Oxford University Press.
Ottoway R N (1980) *Defining the Change Agent.* Unpublished research paper. Manchester University: Department of Management Sciences.
Pearson A (1992) *Nursing at Burford – A Story of Change.* London: Scutari Press.
Peplau H E (1952) *Interpersonal Relationships in Nursing.* New York: Putnam.
Salvage J (1990) The theory and practice of the 'New Nursing'. *Nursing Times,* **86**(4): 42–45.
Turrill T (1985) *Change and Innovation: A Challenge for the NHS.* Management Series 10. London: Institute of Health Services Management.
Wright S G (1989) *Changing Nursing Practice.* London: Edward Arnold.

CHAPTER 3

A History of Nursing Development Units

Alan Pearson

Nursing is essentially a practice, a caring process, which occurs between the nurse and the nursed. Such a reality is inescapable when thinking about nursing's past, present and, most importantly, its future. Since the emergence of modern nursing in the nineteenth century, nurses have pursued a number of different pathways to develop their work and to increase understanding of their role. Florence Nightingale's reforms centred largely on contemporary management theory and on everyday understanding of caring in the sickroom and in public health. As the occupation of nursing developed, greater emphasis was placed on management, training and education and the maintenance of the traditions of the occupation. From the 1920s on, practice itself became decentralised until the late 1950s to early 1960s, when nurses in North America began to develop theoretical constructs of nursing and the practices of nurses began to be studied and valued in Europe and the UK. Alongside this, nurses began to recognise the need for a radical reappraisal of nursing's developmental direction and attempts began to promote innovation in the clinical arena. Different approaches were pursued; the emergence of nursing development units is the present-day continuation of nursing's attempt to develop and reshape itself through innovation.

This chapter traces the historical development of NDUs, including those antecedent to today's designated NDUs. Emphasis is placed on the developments in Oxfordshire and the King's Fund because of my own experience. The term NDU was first adopted in 1981 by a group of nurses working in a small cottage hospital at Burford in Oxfordshire (Swaffield 1982a, Pearson 1983, 1992). The Burford developments were widely discussed in the professional literature and the popular press (for example Alderman 1983, Day 1983,

Follis 1983, Langley 1985, Levi 1985, McIlroy 1985, Swaffield 1982b, 1983c, 1983d, 1983e, 1983f). While this work eventually led to acceptance of the concept in the UK, it was grounded in previous work and occurred alongside a number of other developments which supported it.

Clinical nursing development in the 1960s and 1970s

Until the early 1960s British nursing's major development interests were directed at the management of the nursing service and the education of nurses. The establishment of nursing departments in the universities, notably Edinburgh and Manchester, led to a growing interest in nursing itself – the direct interaction between the nurse and the nursed. It did not take long for these new pockets of influence to generate practical developments in health services. Early developments which aimed at examining, expanding and valuing the way nurses work with patients or clients were exemplified by innovations at the Royal Marsden Hospitals and the Manchester Royal Infirmary. The Royal Marsden – a group of specialist hospitals concerned with cancer care, where Robert Tiffany was the director of nursing – pioneered an all-qualified workforce, the roles of clinical nurse specialist and clinical nurse consultant and an active clinical research programme. The Manchester Royal Infirmary established joint appointments with the department of nursing at the University of Manchester in a designated clinical unit – the Professorial Nursing Unit, led by Professor Baroness McFarlane of Llandaff. Emerging methods of care delivery, such as team nursing, patient allocation and a modified keyworker or primary nursing system, were piloted in both settings. They also pioneered care planning and patient-centred approaches to care (Ashworth and Castledine 1980, Wright 1983).

Much development in the conceptual understanding of nursing occurred in conjunction with these pioneering initiatives. A wealth of literature reflects this. Nursing was making a serious attempt to be clearer about the nature of its practice and its contribution as a discipline in health care. A humanistic approach became dominant and the importance of developing relationships – both between nurses and patients and between nurses and co-health workers – was seen as central to the nursing role.

Growing recognition of the need to reform society's beliefs about the role of women gave rise to a questioning of the subservience of nurses (mainly women) to doctors (mainly men), as well as criticism of the power of medicine by social theorists (Friedson 1975). Nurses began to assert themselves and seek equality within the health care team. Batchelor (1980) lists a number of factors leading to this demand for equality: the changing status of women in society as a whole; the higher status of nurses as reflected by salaries; better qualified applicants to nurse training; more men in senior positions; and the rise in nurses' trade union activity.

Much of this drive for change emanated largely from nurses in national leadership positions and those who became nursing academics in the 1960s. The national nursing bodies exhorted nurses to bring about a radical practice change based on:

- Reorganising work patterns so that care is given by qualified nurses and accountability to the patient is explicit
- Restructuring the nursing team so that the hierarchy is flattened
- Developing a close relationship between nurse and patient, and involvement of the patient in planning care
- Basing practice on a model for nursing which incorporates the concept of holism and clarifies the contribution of nursing to health care and
- The use of a problem-solving approach

The amalgamation of these concepts was said to constitute a major reform in nursing (Pearson and Vaughan 1986) and was referred to as the 'New Nursing' by Salvage (1990).

Similar moves were in process in other countries. The most influential work, in terms of the introduction of NDUs in the UK, was that of Lydia Hall and her colleagues at the Loeb Center for Nursing and Rehabilitation at the Montefiore Hospital and Medical Center in the Bronx, New York. Hall (1966) and Hall et al (1969) argued the case for the provision of hospital beds grouped into units which focus on the delivery of therapeutic nursing; her views were supported by others (e.g. Orem 1966, Alfano 1969, 1971, Poirer 1975, Pearson 1983, 1985, 1987a, 1987b; Pearson et al 1992, Wright 1988). Hall asserted that while patients in acute biological crisis require the services of an acute, high-technology, medically-led unit in the initial phases of hospitalisation, as the crisis lessens the intensity of medical and paramedical intervention also decreases. Both Hall (Hall et al 1975) and her co-worker Alfano (1971) suggested that as the crisis recedes and the need for medical and paramedical intervention falls, the need for rehabilitative, nurturing nursing rises.

They described how the need of post-crisis patients for medical care is rapidly replaced by the need for support, nurturing and teaching once the fear of death and/or pain is resolved. They argued that these latter needs are the legitimate concern of nursing. Based on this reasoning and against a mass of opposition, Lydia Hall established the Loeb Center for Nursing in 1966. An evaluation of its effects on patient outcomes through the conduct of a controlled clinical trial was conducted (Hall et al 1975). This showed that those admitted to the nursing unit, compared to those who pursued a 'normal' patient career in traditional facilities, were readmitted less, were more independent, had a higher post-discharge quality of life and were more satisfied with their experience in hospital. The nursing beds pioneered by Hall are essentially those where 'nursing is the chief therapy and the nurse is the chief therapist' (Tiffany 1977).

The work of Christman (1978, 1988) complemented that of Hall and involved the unification of academic nursing and nursing service at the Rush Medical Center in Chicago. The Chicago development was enormous, funded by the Kellogg Foundation. The college of nursing of the associated university was integrated with the hospital and health service. The Vice President / Nursing – a role similar to a chief nursing officer or executive director of nursing – was also the dean of the college; heads of nursing divisions were heads of departments and professors; charge nurses and staff nurses were also the professors and lecturers of the college. In effect, practice, management, teaching and research were all combined in various nursing roles. The concept was internationally admired and the notion of the unification of these four spheres was well accepted. The development was seen to be exceptional, however, and no widespread replication occurred because of its radical nature and the enormous costs involved. Christman's work, like Hall's, did however influence the future development of nursing and of NDUs. The Royal Marsden and Manchester Royal developments drew on Christman's unification model, though they transformed and refined his ideas into unique approaches.

The evolution of Burford Nursing Development Unit as a prototype NDU also arose from the work of Christman, Hall, McFarlane and Tiffany.

The Burford developments

Under the leadership of Jacqueline Flindall in the 1980s, Oxfordshire Health Authority became committed to the development of clinical nursing and expansion of the nursing role. In 1981, a small community hospital at Burford, in Oxfordshire, was designated as an NDU to explore new approaches to the delivery of nursing care.

Burford Hospital was a nine-bed unit with a traditional style of organising nursing care: nursing was task-oriented rather than professionally-oriented and based on a medical rather than nursing model. Although it served a fairly well-defined geographical area and could have offered a comprehensive service from one site, health visiting and district nursing were in a separate service and had only peripheral links with the hospital.

Burford is a small rural town with a population of 1500. It boasts of having had a hospital for 600 years. A cottage hospital was founded in 1868, and moved to its present site, a building erected through public subscription, in 1902. It became part of the National Health Service in 1948; there had been a number of attempts to close it, on economic and policy grounds, when the centralisation of services on district general hospital sites was prompted in the 1970s. By 1978, medical care was provided by the local general practice of two doctors and the hospital's nine beds had an average occupancy of 85 per cent. A full-time resident matron and 8.5 whole-time-equivalent nurses provided nursing care. There were seven ancillary staff. A 24-hour emergency service for minor injuries was provided and there were outpatient clinics in physiotherapy, chiropody and orthopaedics; 147 outpatients were seen in 1977. An average of four patients spent the day in the hospital each weekday, joining inpatients, in a day-patient service. About 4000 patients were registered with the local medical practice, 730 (17 per cent) of whom were over 65 and 300 (7 per cent) over 75. Of all admissions, 87 per cent were over 65, and 63 per cent were over 75. Most required medical or nursing care to overcome acute problems, holiday relief stays or terminal care. Patients registered with other local practices in neighbouring villages were occasionally admitted, although this was discouraged.

The original cottage hospital had been established by a well-known local doctor and his descendants had continued the link – one of the doctors in post in 1980 was a member of this family. The local people identified with this handing down of a local resource. The matron of 16 years retired in 1980; and after much debate, the health authority decided to recruit a replacement who had the capacity to develop the hospital's nursing service, because the hospital was seen to be uneconomical and its general ethos outdated. I was appointed to this post. From 1981 to 1983 an intensive programme of staff development was introduced for nurses and other members of the clinical team. Radical innovations were successfully introduced and it was established that the unit would primarily provide a professional, 24-hour nursing service. The notion of nursing beds was articulated and developed.

The purpose of the project at Burford was to generate and implement change in nursing and to use a combination of research methods initially to answer the following questions:

1. Could the changes in nursing being advocated by nursing leaders be implemented in an 'ordinary nursing unit'?

2. What effect would such changes have on nurses' and consumers' perceptions of nursing?

3. What effect would the changes have on patient care?

It was also hoped that the project would be able to describe the process of change and the role of the change agent and that it would present hypotheses to be tested as the development progressed.

Answers to these questions were required in order to establish whether the energy needed to implement changes was worth expending and, if it was, in what directions change could be pursued. The open-ended, developmental part of the project was seen to be crucial, because answering only the basic questions would assume that the social setting of nursing was predictable, whereas it was believed that additional hypotheses would soon arise from the project and that testing them would be important. Should the findings demonstrate that advocated changes were of value, it would be shown that it was important to continue with the pursuit of the new ideologies in nursing. The description of the change process and new concepts generated and tested would give direction of other health care teams in planning and implementing changes and might be of use to policy-makers.

An all-qualified nursing team was created between 1981 and 1983 and primary nursing became well established, the nurse acting as keyworker with 24-hour accountability for her patients. Practice came to be based on a nursing model with a clearly defined philosophy of nursing. Nurses worked in partnership with their patients, giving informed choice care which was patient-centred rather than task-centred; individualised care for each patient became the norm.

These innovations in nursing at Burford were regularly described in national nursing journals and newspapers. In one such article it was stated, 'One idea is to use Burford to evaluate properly the different ways of managing care' (Swaffield 1983c). This idea was to become a pilot study, to test the belief that patients benefit from admission to the nursing unit rather than staying in an acute unit. 'Nursing beds – an alternative health care provision' (Pearson et al 1987) is the report of a study to examine the feasibility and effects of establishing nursing beds in the British NHS. Conducted between 1983 and 1985, it was funded by a generous grant from the Monument Trust, enabling three more nursing beds to be situated within the nursing unit.

Outcomes were compared for a group of elderly people who had undergone internal fixation of a fractured neck of femur and were transferred from the acute hospital to Burford, with outcomes for a control group of patients who remained in the acute hospital. The main objective was to establish whether the quality of nursing care in the nursing unit would be at least as good as that in the acute unit and whether the cost of nursing patients in the nursing unit would exceed the cost of nursing similar patients in other hospital wards.

Patients were referred for possible entry into the study by two consultant orthopaedic surgeons and their informed consent was sought. One hundred and seven patients were allocated to a control group and 45 were randomly allocated to the nursing unit. Those in the control group followed the usual course of treatment and remained in the acute hospital, while those allocated to the nursing unit were transferred as soon after surgery as possible. All patients were interviewed three times: on discharge, six weeks later and six months later using a structured interview schedule. On discharge from hospital no significant differences were found between the groups in independence level, patients' expressed satisfaction with hospital care or in life satisfaction score. After six months, dependency had decreased for all groups, with no significant difference between the groups. However, the amount of professional assistance needed by the patient at home in the six months following discharge was twice as much for the control patients as for those patients discharged from the nursing unit. At the six-month interview it was also shown that life satisfaction had increased significantly for those patients admitted to the nursing unit.

Nursing audit scores showed that the quality of nursing differed very significantly between the groups. The quality of nursing was higher and consistently so in the nursing unit. Yet costings showed that nursing patients in the nursing unit incurred no more cost than those in acute beds. No significant difference was found between the groups in total length of stay in NHS care, though patients allocated to the nursing unit spent significantly less time in acute beds.

Although relatively small, the project aroused great interest and support throughout the UK and enabled the research team to explore a larger, major study, with the confidence of having survived the 'mistakes and misconceptions' experienced by many nurse researchers (Hockey 1985).

Meanwhile the Burford service was expanded to incorporate district nursing and health visiting, thus providing a comprehensive nursing and health service to the area. In addition, the unit increasingly organised and conducted in-service training programmes for nurses and other health workers from Oxfordshire, nationwide and even internationally. By 1983, a number of structured educational courses were being offered by Burford NDU in areas such as research, individualised patient care, the management of change and primary nursing. The service to inpatients, outpatients, day patients, the community and patients in their own homes was greatly expanded and costs had been considerably reduced. An evolving research programme and quality assurance strategy was firmly in place.

This first NDU had therefore established a unified approach to practice, research, management and education based in a clinically-oriented unit. The change process and the development of practice within the unit were seen to be successful. Furthermore, the results of the pilot study were extremely positive and suggested that nursing beds could be a useful and effective addition to acute hospital services. However, as the sample size was small and the randomisation technique simple, no concrete conclusions could be drawn: a larger study was needed to validate these preliminary findings. The Burford study therefore became the pilot for a larger study. While the NDU carried on its activities, its team sought funds and support to establish a second unit in a large, city-based acute hospital.

The Oxford Nursing Development Unit

The Oxford NDU was an experimental unit opened in September 1985, funded by a generous grant from one of the Sainsbury Family Charitable Trusts, and strongly supported by the Oxfordshire Health Authority. The nursing unit was the first in the UK to offer the service of 'nursing beds' within an acute general hospital; its philosophy was based on that of Burford NDU and drew on that of the Loeb Center in New York.

The team approached the chief nursing officer of the health authority to seek a suitable site. Three possible sites were offered and the nursing unit was established in an acute general hospital. Six months previously it had been an 18-bed elderly care ward, which had closed owing to financial constraints. The physical layout appeared to have the most potential to create a therapeutic environment. Funding was based on the cost of running 16 nursing beds, plus the cost of refurbishing, data collection and initial staff training. The ward offered one two-bed room, three single rooms and a main area divided into two-bed bays. Lecture rooms and research space were situated nearby.

The new unit had the following aims:

- To admit and care for patients whose primary need was for intensive nursing
- To increase knowledge about the range and effectiveness of different nursing therapies
- To develop forms of nursing which facilitate the involvement of patients as partners and increase their knowledge and control of their own health and
- To teach advanced nursing practice

Primary nursing was chosen as the system for delivering nursing care and was practised in its pure form as described by Manthey (1980). As the unit aimed to provide professional nursing care, to test and generate nursing developments to bring theory and practice more closely together and to serve as a resource and teaching unit, staff selection was of paramount importance. Only qualified nursing staff were employed, registered nurses with a belief in the unit philosophy, a sound clinical background and a good knowledge base.

The patients' day was completely individual, as was their nursing. Patients were encouraged to choose a routine they would normally follow at home, stating what time they wished to have breakfast, bathe and go to bed. Lunch and supper were shared with the two nurses on duty, creating a domestic approach to mealtimes. Nurses and ward orderlies did not wear a uniform, encouraging partnership in care rather than a directive approach. All patients, if able to do so, were taught self-medication. Education and teaching were emphasised, allowing patients to make informed choices in all aspects of their care. All nurses were skilled in massage and aromatherapy, incorporating this into their daily practice. Visiting hours were unrestricted and family participation encouraged.

Referral of patients to the unit was usually recommended by the ward sister or medical officer and approved by the appropriate consultant. In the evaluative phase of the unit, this was restricted to patients with a fractured neck of femur, a cerebral vascular accident or the amputation of a lower limb. Both the senior nurse practitioner and unit medical officer had power of veto on admission to the nursing unit.

Education programmes were an important component of its activities from the outset. Informal and formal courses were offered for local staff and for national and international participants. This was highly successful, attracting many people.

The first patient was admitted to the unit in October 1985. Nursing notes were kept for all patients and audited after discharge by a senior nurse from the department of geriatrics, using the same criteria as the district quality assurance programme (Pearson 1987a). Patients referred to the unit were randomly allocated to a control or treatment group. Those allocated to the control group pursued the usual course of treatment in the acute ward, while those allocated to the treatment group were transferred to the nursing unit as soon as possible. Data were obtained from both groups by personal interview, using the same schedule as in the pilot study, administered by a research assistant. Patients were interviewed on discharge from hospital (within 24 hours whenever possible) and again six weeks and six months after discharge, the last two interviews taking place wherever the patient was then living (their own home, residential accommodation or a nursing home). Data on length of stay and destination on discharge were derived from records.

All social research has limitations by virtue of the fact that its subject is human activity, which is almost by definition individualistic and unpredictable, resisting classification and deductive proof. The Oxford study was no exception and in addition suffered from other known limitations. The study was designed to test the results of the pilot study on a larger sample and one of the problems which soon became apparent was the slow rate of patient referral. Reasons included misunderstanding by nurses about the nature of the study and opposition to the philosophy of nursing underpinning the study from some senior medical staff. Senior nurses from the unit waged a constant propaganda battle with some of their colleagues, but nevertheless the size of the final sample was smaller than hoped. A larger sample would have yielded more information and more reliable evidence.

There was also a loss of data when sample patients had to be withdrawn from the study. This happened if treatment group patients had to be readmitted to the acute hospital or if control patients were discharged before the initial interview and carers felt they could not, at that stage, cope with a visit from a researcher. On principle no patient who wished to withdraw was persuaded to continue and this led to a further small loss of data. (Having said this, a satisfactory response rate of 95.7 per cent was achieved at first interview.)

Problems were also experienced with some of the data collection tools, even though they had already been tested in the pilot study. In particular, the patient service checklist (which originated in the USA) proved difficult to administer, especially at the end of an already long interview. Respondents also sometimes exhibited a natural desire to please (or fear of reprisals?) which may have influenced their answers. This same tendency was sometimes suspected with the life satisfaction index.

The research was based on the assumption that the experience of being nursed in the unit was the dependent variable. This could not, of course, be proved, as many extraneous factors were also at work. In particular it is at least possible that patients' characteristics, habits and life experience may have been at least as effective in promoting (or impeding) recovery as any method of nursing. Even if it were proved that the type of nursing care given to the patient was the dependent variable influencing recovery, there is still the possibility of the Hawthorne effect, by which the special attention paid to study subjects in itself brings about improvement – the process itself becomes the 'cause' of the better outcome.

Finally, there is the question of interviewer bias. All but a tiny fraction of interviews were conducted by the research assistant who was based in the unit. Consistency in data collection and recording was thus reasonably assured, but not interviewer impartiality. As the initial interview nearly always took place before discharge, the interviewer inevitably knew to which group the patient being interviewed belonged – indeed, it was her responsibility to keep track of control group patients who were frequently transferred between wards at the acute hospital or to community hospitals. Awareness of the possibility of bias was the first answer to this problem. The research assistant had previous experience as an interviewer; her training was in social science; and not being a nurse herself, she had few preconceptions about different philosophies of nursing, which minimised the risk of attachment to any one school of thought. Although based in the unit, she did not spend long periods there and, as far as was consistent with good manners, adopted a policy of not becoming involved socially with patients before their discharge.

The sample proved to be totally homogeneous between control and treatment groups in terms of age, sex and living situation before admission to hospital. The important findings of the study (Pearson et al 1988, 1992, Pearson, 1989) are summarised below.

Mortality (death in hospital before initial discharge)

A highly significant difference was found in mortality, with control group patients being three times more likely to die in hospital than treatment group patients. Mortality rates were not a part of the research hypothesis; the finding was surprising and remains unexplained.

Length of stay

Patients randomly allocated to the treatment group were transferred to the nursing unit as soon as possible after acceptance into the study, so it was not unexpected that length of stay in acute care would be lower than the control group, who spent on average three times as long in acute care. Overall, the average length of stay was slightly longer for treatment group patients, but this difference was not significant and does not negate the hypothesis that length of stay in NHS care would be no more for treatment group patients than for those in the control group.

The reasons why patients transferred to the nursing unit should have had longer stays may be linked to their lower dependency scores on discharge. Adequate preparation for discharge, with the patient fully involved in decision-making wherever possible, was part of the philosophy of the unit. This might result in a marginally longer average stay, but a more satisfactory placement on discharge. However, no data were collected about the success of living arrangements after discharge and no conclusions can be drawn about this.

The effect of diagnosis may also be important. The highest average length of stay for all patients was 62.3 days for those who had had amputations in the treatment group, compared to 41.7 days in the control group; but the numbers involved were too small to draw conclusions. The average stay in the nursing unit was longer for patients who had sustained a fracture of the neck of the femur, but shorter for patients with a cerebral vascular accident than for the control group.

Even with the slightly longer average stay recorded at the nursing unit, it is doubtful whether the average total cost would be higher than for patients nursed in community hospitals or acute care beds.

Quality of care

The measure used to assess the quality of nursing care was a nursing audit score; the assumption was made that this would be valid. The results were significantly better for the treatment group, with nearly all scores in the 'excellent' range, whereas the majority of control patients had 'good' or 'satisfactory' scores. Scores were also consistently higher for the treatment group, to a significant degree. Therefore, the quality of nursing care as measured by the nursing audit score was not merely no worse at the nursing unit than on other wards, but was found to be more satisfactory and consistently so, thus supporting the research hypothesis.

Patient service checklist

Another indirect measure of the quality of care was the patient's assessment, as provided by a patient service checklist. Although a tendency to give what was thought to be the 'right' answer had been suspected in the interviews, in the analysis it was proved that treatment group patients were significantly more satisfied with their nursing care, using the checklist, than the control group.

Remarks made by patients at the interview six weeks after discharge tended to support this conclusion. When asked what was good about the nursing received in hospital, 83 per cent of treatment patients, compared to 73 per cent of control patients, gave replies which were graded as 'positive' or 'generally commendatory'. When asked to specify anything about the nursing which was 'not so good' – although less than half of those who replied could do so – three-quarters of the treatment group had no complaints in comparison with just under half of the control patients.

Nursing dependency scores

Nursing dependency on discharge was found to be significantly different for the two groups, with treatment group patients achieving significantly more independence in the activities of daily living than control patients.

This result does not merely support the hypothesis that care in the nursing unit would result in independence levels on discharge no lower than those achieved in other wards. It shows that on average a better result was achieved than for control group patients. Possible reasons for this were discussed above. The fact that differences between the two groups were reduced by the time of the later interviews suggests that it was the input from the nursing unit, motivating patients towards self-care and achieving maximum possible independence, that proved effective. Control group patients remained marginally more dependent six weeks and six months after discharge. Although these differences were not statistically significant, they suggest that where higher independence levels can be achieved in hospital, the improvement can be maintained after discharge.

Life satisfaction scores

Satisfaction with life in general was measured at each interview. The results showed no significant differences either between control and treatment groups or between diagnostic groups. This supported the hypothesis that levels of satisfaction with life in general would be no lower for patients discharged from the nursing unit than for those discharged from other wards.

It is surprising that there was no measurable difference in satisfaction with life between diagnostic groups. Several studies have shown the catastrophic effects on social satisfaction which patients with a stroke often experience. The severe stroke patients in this study faced fundamental changes in their quality of life and expectations for the future; in some cases the interviewer witnessed the process of adjustment which had to be made. These problems were not reflected in lower life satisfaction scores among patients with a cerebral vascular accident, perhaps partly due to loss of data caused by the difficulty of administering the life satisfaction index schedule to dysphasic patients in this group.

Qualitative data on problems after discharge were also of interest here. At the second interview, six weeks after discharge, 65 per cent of treatment patients admitted to problems compared to 57 per cent of control patients, and similar results were obtained after six months. Yet there was no significant difference in life satisfaction scores between the two groups at either interview. Patients in the nursing unit were encouraged to verbalise their problems and were not discouraged from expressing negative feelings; this openness may have helped them to cope with ongoing problems while still maintaining a reasonable level of life satisfaction.

In general, results from the quantitative data analysis were more consistent across the board for treatment patients than for the control group. The standard deviation in all areas of quantitative measurement was notably lower for treatment patients, a group who had all experienced care in one nursing unit with a cohesive philosophy underpinning the delivery of nursing care, whereas control patients had been nursed in various wards in different hospitals. This may partly account for the difference, but is hardly adequate as a complete explanation of such a striking result. No other factor provides a more satisfactory explanation than the effect of exposure to the style of nursing practised in the nursing unit.

Qualitative data inevitably yield less rigorous results than data which are amenable to statistical analysis. Nevertheless such data contribute to the total picture by adding depth and richness to the bare outline provided by quantifiable data. This group of patients emerged as generally tolerant, usually uncomplaining and reluctant to criticise their experience of health care generally and of nursing in particular. They placed great value on nurses' personal qualities of kindness and friendliness, more so than on their technical skills, but tended to remember little of the advice they had been given, except in very general terms. Nurses were perceived as very busy people and specific criticisms of staff shortage were made by patients in both groups.

Treatment group patients were almost twice as likely as control group patients to remember being given advice in hospital about their convalescence (42 per cent treatment, 23 per cent control); specifically, advice on 'taking care' and taking exercise was reported by 20 per cent in the treatment group but only 5 per cent in the control group. They were less likely to be critical of the nursing care they had received; only 32 per cent of treatment patients compared to 58 per cent of the control group made general or specific complaints. They were more likely to admit to problems six weeks after discharge (65 per cent treatment, 33 per cent control), but after six months this difference was less apparent. Problems were similar for both groups: health and mobility problems, psychological problems and miscellaneous personal, practical and financial problems were reported at second and third interviews by both groups. At the six-month interview of patients with cerebral vascular accident, health problems were particularly prominent for treatment group patients, while a higher proportion of control patients reported psychological problems.

A small minority of younger treatment group patients had experienced boredom and depression in the nursing unit, complaining of lack of stimulus because of the age and dependency of fellow patients and the lack of recreational facilities. More typically, however, patients who had experienced care at the nursing unit were complimentary, expressing cordial feelings of appreciation at the 'homely', 'family' atmosphere. 'Although I was ill,' said one, 'I quite enjoyed it.' Similar sentiments were noted in the control group from three patients who had been nursed at a community hospital.

Overall findings

In summary, the results suggest that in a homogeneous sample of patients, differences between control and treatment group patients have emerged which are the effect of the operation of the dependent variable – i.e. therapeutic nursing care at the nursing unit. Five of the study hypotheses were supported and the data strongly suggest that the nursing unit was successful in promoting recovery, increasing quality and conserving costs, as follows:

1. Care in the nursing unit will be no worse than that provided by other wards.

This was supported by nursing audit scores. Quality of care as judged by these scores was found to be significantly higher – and more consistently so – in the nursing unit than in other wards.

2. Care in the nursing unit will result in an independence level no lower than that achieved in other wards.

This was supported by the nursing dependency scores. Not only were these scores lower than those of patients cared for in other hospital wards, they were significantly so in patients who were cared for in the nursing unit when they were discharged from hospital.

3. Patients discharged from the nursing unit will be no less satisfied with the nursing care received than patients in other wards.

This was supported by the patient service checklist scores and the qualitative data obtained. Indeed, the patient service checklist scores were significantly higher in patients who were cared for in the nursing unit and there were fewer complaints about care in nursing unit patients six weeks after discharge than in control group patients. Satisfaction with care was therefore higher in nursing unit patients.

4. Patients discharged from the nursing unit will have a level of satisfaction with life in general no lower than that of patients discharged from other wards.

This was supported by life satisfaction scores, which were not significantly different between control and treatment groups.

5. Readmission rates for patients discharged from the nursing unit will be no higher than those for patients discharged from other wards.

This hypothesis could not be tested because of insoluble problems in collecting these data.

6. Length of stay and/or cost per patient should be no longer/ higher than for patients nursed on other wards.

This was supported by a significantly shorter average stay in the acute hospital for treatment group patients. The total length of stay in an NHS bed was not significantly different between groups. Treatment group patients incurred lower average costs than those in the control group.

Thus five of the six hypotheses were supported by the research findings and the remaining hypothesis could neither be supported nor refuted because of lack of data. In addition, significantly fewer treatment group patients died in hospital; significantly more were discharged to their own homes; and the results of the quantitative data were more consistent for treatment group patients, with smaller standard deviations for most factors of analysis.

The findings therefore strongly indicate that nursing bed care has a positive effect on recovery, quality, satisfaction and mortality, which supports the study assumption that nursing in itself is a therapeutic force. Contemporary health care planners and policy-makers explicitly and consistently urge higher quality, better outcomes and lower costs: this study clearly demonstrated that nursing beds can achieve all three objectives. Such strong results highlighted the need to maintain the experimental unit and to replicate it in other areas of the NHS. The findings of this study clearly demonstrated the quantitative and qualitative benefits of providing the therapeutic nursing in a designated nursing unit where nursing was the primary therapy and nurses were the chief therapists.

In the event, however, the Oxford NDU was closed by the Oxfordshire Health Authority in 1989 and, despite later assurances that the unit would be revived, it has never reopened. Why this occurred is still unexplained. Pembrey and Punton (1990) suggest that it may have been due to a lack of integration of the unit with the wider hospital, but this explanation is purely speculative. The unit challenged the status quo and questioned the legitimacy of existing power structures; it also gained much positive publicity and this may have led opponents to gather support for its closure.

Tameside Nursing Development Unit

While Burford NDU was being established in 1981, other work was starting at Tameside General Hospital in Ashton-under-Lyne. This began with a focus on the joint appointment concept and was based in an aged care unit of the district general hospital. As at Burford, the emphasis was on the generation of change within nursing and health care, stemming from analysis and action in and of practice itself (Wright 1989a). This led to a series of innovations in elderly care – the dismantling of routine and depersonalising practices, primary nursing and the involvement of patients in planning and managing their own daily lives. By 1985, the Tameside project was well recognised and was the subject of much publicity in the professional and general press. It was named the Tameside Nursing Development Unit in 1985 and was firmly established as a centre of clinical excellence involved in practice, teaching, research and development.

The NDU leader, Steve Wright, pursued further development on the nature and contribution of NDUs (Wright 1989a, 1989b) and worked closely with nursing leaders, power-holders and policy-makers in the health service and government to promote the NDU concept in the UK. An evaluation of the Tameside unit was funded by the Department of Health. By 1991, staff of the unit were in constant demand for assistance from other organisations at home and abroad, and The European Nursing Development Agency (TENDA) was established in 1992 to service these demands.

The King's Fund Centre Nursing Developments Programme

In 1988, the King's Fund Centre for Health Services Development established a new programme to pursue clinical nursing development, led by Jane Salvage. Given the success of the Burford, Oxford and Tameside units, and increasing interest in their approaches to changing and developing nursing practice, the programme was focused on piloting more NDUs and setting up a national NDU network and a primary nursing network. Jane Salvage had already investigated the emergence of the three early NDUs (Salvage 1989a, 1989b, 1990), and the King's Fund programme was to have a significant effect on the future development of NDUs across the UK. Funding from the Sainsbury Family Charitable Trusts was used by the King's Fund to pump-prime the setting up of four full NDUs in clinical units with a desire to become centres for practice development and in health authorities where support was apparent. A further 20 embryonic units were awarded small seeding grants to foster their growth. The NDU network linked these units with each other to provide support and to share ideas.

A survey I carried out in 1991 (Pearson 1993) suggested that the network initiative was very successful. Among the 70 groups that initially expressed an interest in joining the NDU network, 52 completed and returned a postal questionnaire, resulting in a response rate of 74 per cent. Forty-four per cent of the respondents had attended one or more of the NDU network conferences and over half found them very or quite helpful. Among those that had not attended any conference, 'didn't know about them' was the main reason given. About two-fifths of the respondents had attended study days or workshops organised by other NDUs and none reckoned that they were of no help. Twenty-two respondents had private meetings with Jane Salvage and/or Gill Black, the King's Fund NDU project worker, and 86 per cent regarded these meetings as very or quite helpful. Sixty per cent had previously made telephone contact or corresponded with Nursing Developments Programme staff from the King's Fund Centre, and the vast majority found this of substantial help.

Among the 52 respondents, 28 were associated with or working in an NDU and 18 of the questionnaires were completed by the clinical leader of the NDU. Of the 28 NDUs, 63 per cent had fewer than 30 beds or client caseload and 15 per cent had over 100. Sixty per cent of the units were located in general acute hospitals, 11 per cent in community hospitals and 11 per cent in specialist units. Twenty-four of the NDUs were recognised as an NDU by one or more of the following bodies – health authority, district general manager, unit general manager and director of nursing services. Of the four units which had no recognition from any of the above bodies, all were working towards recognition as an NDU.

Regarding the organisational structure which supported the NDU, 39 per cent belonged to part of the traditional health service structure, 46 per cent to an outside structure and the rest were part of a new structure. In total, 36 per cent of the NDUs received additional resources from their organisations, mainly in the form of additional finance.

Sixty-four per cent of the NDUs reported that they received a great deal or some assistance from the King's Fund Nursing Developments Programme. Eighty-two and 52 per cent received little or no help from the regional health authority or district health authority. District or unit general managers gave 63 per cent of these units a great deal of or some assistance. Nurses in the NDUs offered considerably more assistance to the NDU than nurse managers, nurse educators, nurse academics or doctors.

Nearly 90 per cent of the NDUs were undertaking evaluation of their units or of specific aspects of nursing practice, mainly in the form of piloting innovations; five NDUs had fully funded evaluative studies in progress.

The two events most often identified as seminal in the NDUs' establishment or development were the introduction of specific changes and new methods of organising care. Other relatively common answers were the creation of a change agent role in the unit, the evolutionary process and the development of an agreed philosophy.

The 28 NDUs were asked about the most difficult obstacles to developing their units. 'Staff motivation, frustration and attrition' was the most common answer. Organisational changes outside the NDU's control were perceived as a major obstacle, as was the availability of resources (funding, expertise).

The most important feature of an NDU was identified as 'development and change'. The umbrella term included the following answers: being a centre for change in breadth and depth, advancing nursing practice and providing staff development. The second most common answer was 'carrying out research and evaluation'. The characteristic of an NDU to act as a standard or role model was recognised by many as essential.

Units which had tried but failed to establish an NDU were asked about their perceived obstacles. Lack of money was the major one.

In addition, lack of support from managers, senior nurses or other personnel and lack of knowledge were often cited.

The Department of Health was closely involved with this expansion of the NDU concept and was aware of the success of the King's Fund NDU network. In 1991, the government allocated £3 million to establish further NDUs, a major programme to be managed by the King's Fund. By 1993, over 70 NDUs were active in the UK; Barbara Vaughan had taken over as director of King's Fund programme; and NDUs had become well-established components of the health system.

NDUs in other countries

NDUs as such did not emerge in North America and there is none as yet in continental Europe, although there is much interest there. In Australia, two professorial nursing units, based on the work at Burford and Oxford, but more formally linked to a university faculty of nursing, were established in Geelong, Victoria, in 1987 (Pearson and Baker 1992, Baker and Pearson 1992). I headed these units as professor of nursing and they generated an interest in NDUs across Australia. While no organised, planned approach to the establishment of clinical units to develop nursing has yet emerged, there is increasing interest in the concept and the Geelong units are still in place. A new unit opened in 1993 at Flinders Medical Centre in Adelaide, South Australia.

This chapter has surveyed the establishment and growth of NDUs in the UK and elsewhere. Although these units have drawn on the thinking of nurses from other countries, they are a unique, British concept which characterises the emphasis of British nursing on the practical application of new ideas to patient care. The units have already turned around much of the rigid thinking of nursing's past and have generated a climate for change which will help nursing to rethink its place in the health system, and thus to build plans for a strong future. Other chapters in this book elaborate further on nursing's visions for the future and on the contributions NDUs have made, and will continue to make, to this process.

References

Alderman C (1983) Individual care in action. *Nursing Times*, 19 January: 15–17.

Alfano G J (1969) A professional approach to nursing practice. *Nursing Clinics of North America* **4**(3): 487–493.

Alfano G J (1971) Healing or caretaking – Which will it be? *Nursing Clinics of North America* **6**: 273–280.

Ashworth P and Castledine G (1980) Joint service-education appointments in nursing. *Medical Teacher* **2**(6): 295–299.

Baker H and Pearson A (1992) *The Subjective Experience of Admission to a Nursing Unit: An Interpretive Study.* Deakin Institute of Nursing Research: Research Paper Number 6. Geelong: Deakin University Press.

Batchelor I (1980) *The Multidisciplinary Clinical Team – A Working Paper.* London: King's Fund.

Christman L (1978) Nursing practice, whose responsibility? *Australian Nurses Journal* **8**(2): 37–41, 61.

Christman L (1988) A conceptual model for centres of excellence in nursing. *Nursing Administration Quarterly* **12**(4): 1–4.

Day J (1983) The little hospital making a big impact in health care. *Witney Gazette.*

Follis P (1983) More autonomy for nurses in Burford's new 'Care Charter'. *BMA News Review*, September: ii-iv.

Friedson E (1975) *The Profession of Medicine.* New York: Dodds, Mead & Co.

Hall L E (1966) Another View of Nursing Care and Quality. In M Straub and K Parker (eds) *Continuity of Patient Care: The Role of Nursing.* Washington, DC: Catholic University of America Press.

Hall L E, Rifkin E and Levine H (1969) The Loeb Center for Nursing and Rehabilitation, Montefiore Hospital and Medical Center, Bronx, New York. *International Journal of Nursing Studies* **6**: 81–95.

Hall L E, Alfano G J, Rifkin E and Levine H S (1975) *Longitudinal Effects of an Experimental Nursing Process.* New York: Loeb Center for Nursing.

Hockey L (1985) *Nursing Research: Mistakes and Misconceptions.* Edinburgh: Churchill Livingstone.

Langley W (1985) The hospital that threw out the rules. *Daily Mail*, 31 October.

Levi P (1985) Hospital life can be just what the patient orders. *Daily Telegraph*, 6 November.

Manthey M (1980) *The Practice of Primary Nursing.* Oxford: Blackwell Scientific Publications.

McIlroy F (1985) Nursing which gives patients a say is extended. *Daily Telegraph*, 25 October.

Orem D E (1966) Discussion of paper by L E Hall: Another View of Nursing Care Equality. In M Straub and K Parker (eds) *Continuity of Patient Care: The Role of Nursing.* Washington, DC: Catholic University of America Press.

Pearson A (1983) *The Clinical Nursing Unit.* London: Heinemann.

Pearson A (1985) *The Effects of Introducing New Norms into a Nursing Unit and an Analysis of the Process of Change.* Unpublished PhD thesis, Department of Social Science, University of London, Goldsmiths College.

Pearson A (ed.) (1987a) *Primary Nursing: Nursing in the Burford and Oxford Nursing Development Units.* London: Croom Helm.

Pearson A (ed.) (1987b) *Nursing Quality Measurement – Quality Assurance*

Methods for Peer Review. Chichester: John Wiley.

Pearson A (1989) Therapeutic Nursing – Transforming Models and Theories in Action. In J Akinsanya (ed.) *Recent Advances in Nursing.* London: Longman.

Pearson A (1992) *Nursing at Burford: A Story of Change.* London: Scutari.

Pearson A (1993) *An Evaluation of the King's Fund Nursing Development Unit Network.* In press.

Pearson A and Baker H (1992) *Quality of Care: Do Contemporary Nursing Approaches Make a Difference?* Deakin Institute of Nursing Research: Research Paper Number 5. Geelong: Deakin University Press.

Pearson A and Vaughan B (1986) *Nursing Models for Practice.* London: Heinemann.

Pearson A, Durand I and Punton S (1988) The feasibility and effectiveness of nursing beds. *Nursing Times (Occasional Paper)* **84**(47): 48–50.

Pearson A, Punton S and Durand I (1992) *Nursing Beds: An Evaluation of Therapeutic Nursing.* London: Scutari Press.

Pearson A, Smith A, Punton S and Durand I (1987) *Nursing Beds – An Alternative Health Care Provision.* Unpublished.

Pembrey S and Punton S (1990) The lessons of nursing beds. *Nursing Times* **86**(14): 44–45.

Poirer B (1975) Loeb Center: What nursing can and should be. *The American Nurse* **7**(1): 5.

Salvage J (ed.) (1989a) Nursing developments. *Nursing Standard* **3**(22): 25–28.

Salvage J (1989b) Building centres of excellence. *Nursing Standard* **3**(48): 53–56.

Salvage J (1990) The theory and practice of the 'New Nursing'. *Nursing Times (Occasional Paper)* **84**(4): 42–45.

Swaffield L (1982a) Spanner in the works. *Nursing Times,* 23 June: 1049–1054.

Swaffield L (1982b) Quality of life. *Nursing Times,* 10 November: 325–328.

Swaffield L (1983c) A model for the future. *Nursing Times,* 12 January: 13–16.

Swaffield L (1983d) Change for the better. *Nursing Times,* 20 April: 58–61.

Swaffield L (1983e) The art of not knowing best. *Nursing Times,* 6 July: 14.

Swaffield L (1983f) A commitment to change. *Nursing Times,* 3 August: 14.

Tiffany C H (1977), *Nursing Organizational Structure and the Real Goals of Hospitals: A Correlational Study.* Unpublished PhD Thesis, Indiana University.

Wright S G (1983) The best of both worlds. *Nursing Times* **79**(42): 25–29.

Wright S G (1988) Developing nursing – The contribution to quality. *International Journal of Health Care Quality Assurance* **1**(1): 12–18.

Wright S G (1989a) *Changing Nursing Practice.* London: Edward Arnold.

Wright S G (1989b) Defining the nursing development unit. *Nursing Standard* **4**(7): 29–31.

CHAPTER 4

Greenhouses, Flagships and Umbrellas

Jane Salvage

What is a nursing development unit? Working for the King's Fund Centre's Nursing Developments Programme, my colleagues and I were always being asked this question, and we had a pat answer: 'A nursing development unit is a care setting which aims to achieve and promote excellence in nursing.' Yet this is more a description than a definition, and a rather dry one at that, so we frequently found ourselves searching for a suitable way of expressing what we meant more intuitively and vividly. At various times NDUs were likened to greenhouses (protected environments to nurture the delicate seedlings of clinical practice development), umbrellas (to shelter a variety of activities), flagships (to proclaim the value of nursing) and laboratories (where a range of innovations could be tested and refined).

All those analogies capture something of the essence of NDUs, but not the whole. Their variety reflects the complexity and richness of NDUs rather than any lack of agreement or clarity about what they are. The images also illustrate the human dimension: an NDU is not bricks and mortar so much as a focus for a dynamic process of human endeavour, easier to recognise when seen or experienced than it is to define. Teams of nurses in hospital or community who believe they are working towards NDU ideals are free to use the NDU title if they wish, as no one can claim copyright of it. Conversely, there are many units functioning effectively as NDUs which do not use the title. Others – far fewer – may call themselves NDUs but do not yet display the characteristics which are generally regarded as essential NDU features.

Earlier chapters in this book have explored some of the roots of the NDU movement. It is important to describe these, not only as a matter of debate and record but for the light they shed on the issue

51

of definition. The trends and traditions from which NDUs have evolved all contribute to the special identity and characteristics of these pioneering units; understanding where they are coming from should help to clarify what they are. Everyone involved in the movement naturally has his or her own, unique view, so a major issue we faced in trying to take the work forward was to establish a consensus on what an NDU is – and is not!

The question of definition is not simply an academic one. As interest in NDUs grew, the apparently simple task of agreeing a definition turned out to be highly charged. As with any fashionable new idea, the issue of ownership soon came to the fore, especially as it was linked with the possibility of funding and legitimation from the King's Fund. The challenge to us, even when it was only implicit, was unmistakable: what right had we to impose our definition or model? Who did we think we were? Yet this process of debate and definition was a valuable one, since it obliged all of us working together on NDUs to sharpen our thinking and to learn how to deal constructively with the disagreement and doubt it provoked on the way.

Why the NDU movement has emerged

Table 4.1 summarises my own perspective on the trends in society, health care and nursing from which the NDU movement springs. (It makes an interesting comparison with Pearson's analysis in Chapter 3.) At its simplest, the movement can be described as an attempt to improve patient care by developing nurses and nursing. Although nursing is one of the most costly items in the NHS budget and nurses give 90 per cent of direct professional health care, nursing generally has remained low on the management agenda at the national and local level. According to the policy analysts Beardshaw and Robinson (1990), 'the challenge will be to reshape nursing – and equip nurses – to deliver the most effective care possible in the coming decade.' NDUs are a direct response to that challenge.

Good nursing is indisputably important to patients in hospital and in the community, especially as it is increasingly clear that it not only makes patients more comfortable mentally and physically, but plays an active role in preventing ill health, restoring them to health and enabling them to achieve their maximum potential. Yet this key contribution to health care has been sorely neglected. There has been inadequate investment in the development of nursing and nurses, so staff often lack the skills, education or opportunity to

Social trends	Health care trends	Nursing trends
1970s		
Feminism	Trade unionism,	Professionalism
Consumerism	collectivism	American
Belief in personal growth,	Better professional	influence
New Age ideas	education	Homegrown
Small is beautiful		Pressure for
		reform
1980s		
Managerialism	Management culture	Expanding
Coping with chaos	Dissatisfaction with	knowledge
High tech	medical dominance	Clinical
Monetarism	Patients' rights	leadership
Swing to right	Low morale	Publications
	Cost-consciousness	Conferences
	Attacks on NHS	The New Nursing
		Disillusionment
		'Crisis'
1990s		
'High touch' is back	Value for money	Nurse-led
	Focus on outcomes	initiatives

NURSING DEVELOPMENT UNITS

Table 4.1 The genesis of the NDU movement: some contributory factors

acquire new expertise, to scrutinise their work or to introduce changes which may benefit patients.

On the plus side, there is now an upsurge of interest in nursing and midwifery practice which has both influenced and been influenced by the emergence of NDUs. Positive measures include first steps towards a career structure which rewards experience and responsibility in clinical work; major growth in nursing research; and significant improvements in the quality and availability of basic and continuing education. Many obstacles to progress remain, including declining recruitment, inability to retain staff, lack of funds and resistance to change among nurses and their medical and management colleagues. Only a profession that is open, dynamic and questioning will retain public and staff confidence: real, lasting improvements in practice will only be achieved through the continuing development and support of all nursing staff. This is where NDUs come in.

For me the foundation stone of the NDU movement is its value base. The work of the units and of the development agencies which support them is built on a set of values which emphasises respect for each human being. Each patient/client and each staff member has an equal right to be treated as an individual, to have their choices and preferences upheld wherever possible. Mission statements such as this are becoming common in nursing; the point about an NDU is that lip-service is not enough and that these values are the touchstone, not only for setting the unit's goals but for how it tries to achieve them. This means not only that care must be genuinely patient-centred, but that everyone's contribution, from sister to auxiliary, must be valued and their opinions sought and heeded.

Another key belief is that people are naturally creative and effective even though their abilities may have been curtailed or blocked by their life experiences. This optimistic view of human nature assumes that personal growth is possible for everyone and that the right kind of development/training can help us to release our blocked potential. Personal growth is also an essential element in organisational change (which is the business of an NDU) and one way of achieving positive change is to develop people's effectiveness and ability to plan, manage and respond to it. This focus on growth is relevant to everyone: project leaders, all other staff and patients. Successfully managing the change which ill health brings to your life is a major challenge for patients; nurses can help them handle it through developing their own skills and creating a more supportive and facilitative patient care environment.

The nursing developments team I headed at the King's Fund Centre, which plays a central role in supporting and promoting NDUs, is fortunate to be part of an organisation which values its staff and actively encourages their development. While working with nurses to help them establish their NDUs, we also concentrate on our own personal and professional growth, individually and as a team. We are not telling other people 'how to do it' in the traditional expert/client way, but sharing with our working partners our own experience of the processes which they too are undergoing.

A second formative influence on the King's Fund approach to NDUs has been our understanding of the need to manage change effectively and our growing ability to do this. Theories of change and development are often discussed in health care today and in society as a whole; paperbacks on them can even be bought at railway station bookstalls – always a barometer of social trends. Like all theories, change theories take their direction from their value base; those that guide our approach to NDUs flow from the positive view of human beings outlined above.

We espouse the idea that the journey to change is as important as the destination and practise a step-by-step approach, emphasising the importance of preparation and forethought and of acknowledging how we feel as well as what we think about the process. In today's global and health care environment, change is not a one-off event but a way of life. The NDU is constantly involved in change of some kind and attempts to direct it effectively by working in a cycle, which incorporates sharing a philosophy and a commitment, setting goals, celebrating successes, offering ongoing support and undertaking regular progress reviews. In clarifying this approach, our team was helped enormously by working on our own professional and personal development with independent consultants, especially Robin Coates and Sue Coates.

The theory and practice of change in organisations has been tested and refined in many health care settings, including the King's Fund Centre's other fieldwork as well as NDUs. This enables us to draw on earlier research and experience of work-based schemes for developing health services. A rich and stimulating literature is emerging on this within nursing and we were also able to consider the perspectives offered by King's Fund colleagues including David Towell (Towell and Harries 1979) and Barbara Stocking (Stocking 1985).

Discussing our work with non-nursing colleagues engaged in similar projects, but in different fields, has been invaluable. At the King's Fund Centre this included projects on informal carers, mental health service users and organisational audit. Many of the complexities and problems of this type of change work are universal and we often talk about the need to avoid reinventing the wheel, but in a true learning process which involves our emotions as well as our intellects (Towell's 'innovation from within') it is sometimes necessary to tread the same path which others have already trod. Studies of other projects may mean little until we have minted the experience freshly for ourselves; it is then reassuring to read them again and find out that many of our difficulties arose from the nature of the work rather than our own ineptitude.

This growth of interest and expertise in health services development has been a significant influence on our work. Pilot projects such as NDUs are gaining credibility as a means of testing in practice the bright ideas of policy-makers or practitioners. They encourage a two-way process: policy-makers and analysts can see how well their ideas actually work, while practitioners, user groups and others can attempt to influence the policy agenda by demonstrating the effectiveness of their local approaches. Development projects offer a way of bridging the top-down/bottom-up divide, as they embody the strategic link between the two.

Social scientists have provided much insight into this type of social experiment. Human enterprises such as health care systems are characterised by a multitude of influences and by the normal muddle of everyday life, and projects which attempt to reproduce the controlled conditions of the laboratory find themselves shaped by unpredictable or uncontrollable variables. NDUs do not set out to be experiments of that kind and it is therefore difficult to 'prove' that Innovation X led to Outcome Y – although these are the causal links which governments and economists demand. Development projects may come up with what seem to be authoritative solutions to specific problems and this is a major focus of their work, as their solutions may then be adopted elsewhere. Equally important, though, is their role in demonstrating what processes or ways of working can motivate staff and build a climate in which creativity flourishes. Outcomes are their overriding concern (how does nursing make a difference?), but they also aim to deepen understanding of how good results can be achieved. What can be disseminated to other units is knowledge of the development process itself, as well as specific, tried and tested innovations, for without expert management of the change process the innovation is unlikely to stick.

Another key perspective on NDUs is their mission to put into practice the ideals of the 'New Nursing' movement. (Alan Pearson once described the work of the Oxford NDU as 'the contemporary ideology of nursing in action'.) The driving force of the New Nursing, a reform from within the profession, is the desire to replace the prevailing occupational model, the bureaucratic one, with a professional model which has the skilled, knowledgeable practitioner as its linchpin. Empowering the nurse to practise as an autonomous professional, it is argued, will help her to empower the patients with whom she works in partnership. While these contentions are open to debate (Salvage 1992), the proponents of the New Nursing are undoubtedly a major force in British nursing and provide high-profile clinical leadership which has long been lacking. Many of these leaders are closely involved with NDUs.

NDUs are therefore an important vehicle for testing these ideas and ideals and for strengthening the clinical nursing knowledge base. They open up a variety of interlinked issues which must all be tackled if nursing is to play a full part in modern health care. The practice of nursing is currently undervalued by nurses themselves, by doctors, by managers and by politicians: NDUs provide living, breathing exemplars of what can be achieved when nurses win the freedom and the resources to use and extend their expertise.

A final factor which has assisted the birth of NDUs is the so-called nursing crisis. Whenever the British media in the late 1980s mentioned nursing, it was almost invariably to warn of the impending health care crisis precipitated by shortages of staff. Demographic trends, low morale and low pay were all frequently cited as reasons why fewer recruits were coming into the occupation and qualified staff were leaving it. Whether the crisis was really new or a history of neglect exacerbated by current problems is beside the point; the crisis talk provided an opportunity to advocate new solutions such as NDUs. They offer realistic and pragmatic ways of tackling complex issues such as measuring cost-effectiveness or raising morale, and this helps nurses to persuade managers and policy-makers to support the new units politically and financially.

Next steps in developing the NDU model

These, then, were some of the experiences, trends and ideas in which the NDU movement took root. They were taken up in many places by different people. How did the King's Fund contribute? Early in 1988 I was appointed director of the newly created Nursing Developments Programme at the King's Fund Centre for Health Services Development in London. The programme was created in response to the Fund's awareness of the need for clinical nursing development and its concern at the current nursing 'crisis'. My remit was to focus on clinical practice development in nursing, midwifery and health visiting, within the framework of values held by the Centre and articulated in its mission statement. I had a free hand to develop the programme and the prospect of funding from the Sainsbury Family Charitable Trusts.

In deciding how to make the best use of these considerable resources, I was strongly influenced by the good nursing practice I had seen during my previous work as a nursing journalist and teacher. All over the UK, in every branch of nursing and its sister professions, I saw wonderful examples of nursing at its best: innovative, creative and humane. Yet only a handful of these achievements were ever written up in the professional press or described at conferences and their leaders were often self-effacing and seemingly unaware of how good their work was (sometimes confiding that no one had ever before taken an interest in what they were doing). I also visited settings such as Oxford, Burford, Tameside and the Royal Marsden Hospitals which were already a byword for nursing excellence and whose leaders had become skilled at using the media to share their experiences and raise their profile. What I saw made me ask two questions: What, if anything, did all these places have in common which set them apart from the average? And if their shared recipe for success could be identified, would it be possible to teach other nurses how to use it?

Their success in developing clinical nursing excellence seemed to depend partly on how well they were rooted in the specific context of their host organisation and how well they identified and responded to the particular needs of their organisation and its clients. Inevitably each unit, ward or clinic had its own characteristics and identity. They also shared certain features, however – the main ingredients of the recipe we wanted to describe and test in the NDU programme:

1. The unit is based in the clinical setting (ward, clinic or community team) where care is given. It may have close links with other units or institutions such as research and higher education, but it is a normal functioning part of mainstream health care provision. Any kind of setting where nursing is practised is appropriate (community, psychiatry, intensive care, etc.), though more experience is needed to determine whether certain kinds of setting or specialty are more suited than others to successful development of units adopting the King's Fund NDU model.

2. The unit begins life as a small, focused project on a ward or within a team. Eventually, it undertakes outreach work beyond this base, but only when its identity, way of working and change process are firmly established, which may take months or years depending on the unit's initial strengths. Exceptions to this may occur when a whole hospital or neighbourhood embarks on a planned change programme, but this seems relatively rare in nursing.

3. The unit must be, and must be seen to be, led and owned by clinical nurses. This requires good clinical nursing leadership from the outset, the delegation of decision-making to the lowest

possible level and continuing participation by all nursing staff.

4. The unit's approach to change is built on strong practitioner involvement and a democratic management style. The aim is to work in partnership with managers and other professionals, with nurses acting and recognised as equals in the team. For this reason it is crucial that units initiate or volunteer themselves to participate in change programmes, rather than being selected by senior managers. Similarly, the units must demonstrate that they are already ripe for change; a development project of this type is not designed to be a remedial measure for problem wards or teams.

5. The unit's focus is developing nursing practice. The improvement of nursing education, research and management may also occur (and usually does), but practice must be the core. Inevitably, this encourages nurses to engage in dialogue with doctors and others on clinical issues, but the focus on nursing is its reason for existence and must remain clear and undiluted.

6. Staff development in the widest sense, to encourage personal and organisational growth, is the foundation of lasting progress. The unit therefore devotes human and financial resources to staff development, including designated time. Such activity is recognised as an indispensable element of nursing work, not as a luxury or an add-on.

From these common characteristics we could begin to define a nursing development unit. Based in a care setting which aims to achieve and promote excellence in nursing, it is committed to improving patient care by maximising the therapeutic potential of nursing; nurses work in partnership with a health care team in which the patient is the key member. In a climate where each person's contribution is valued and an open, questioning, supportive approach is fostered, certain activities are essential to the unit's mission (Table 4.2).

- Offering the best possible standards of care.
- Monitoring the quality of care and taking appropriate follow-up action.
- Evaluating the effects of the unit's activity on patients and staff.
- Enabling nurses to develop, personally and professionally.
- Sharing knowledge and experience with a wider audience.

Table 4.2 Key activities of an NDU

The staff of each NDU may also agree on additional key features specific to their unit; for example, see Wright (1989) on Tameside NDU. Within the overall framework there is enormous room for diversity.

Setting up new NDUs

This was the focus we needed for the new nursing developments programme. We would test the recipe by selecting a small number of actual/potential NDUs for pump-priming grants and development input. Over the three-year development phase we would help them to work towards mutually agreed goals. These would be specific objectives designed to realise the multifaceted aspirations of each NDU: to act as a demonstration or pilot site for nursing innovation; to be a test-bed for specific initiatives; to be a powerhouse for clinical practice development; to provide clinical leadership; to focus on developing nurses in order to develop nursing; and in sum, to be a flagship for nursing.

The King's Fund Centre was a perfect home for the programme in many ways, with its rich store of experience of project work across the spectrum of health and social care and its growing expertise in managing the process of change and empowering service users and direct care providers. This multidisciplinary, client-centred approach was a valuable counterbalance to the introversion of nursing. Moreover, the Fund's aura of authority and expertise was invaluable, as was its political and philosophical independence (as distinct from neutrality). All this and funding without strings but with wise support – it seemed almost too good to be true.

The next step was to develop a more detailed strategy. Working together with nursing leaders (especially those from existing NDUs) and Fund colleagues, we searched for a way to make the NDU vision achievable. We wanted to make a big impact with resources which, while generous, would vanish without trace if they were spread too thinly across the huge nursing workforce. After agreeing that we would focus on exploring the potential of NDUs as a means of improving patient care, we needed practical tools, starting with processes and criteria for project selection.

From the outset we were clear that NDUs were not the only or necessarily the best strategy for nursing development. Encouraging nurses to establish NDUs did not mean that other approaches were not equally valid or fruitful – indeed, bringing about change in a field as large and diverse as nursing requires a whole range of development strategies. We had chosen one with potential and were committed to exploring it in a supportive but critical way, so for good or ill we put most of our eggs in that basket. To explore it effectively, a 'model' had to be constructed and then tested in practice. Elements of it could already be found in the existing NDUs and similar sites, but further refinement and specification was needed as a basis for selection and testing in the field.

The refinement of the model was a surprisingly sensitive issue and stirred up strong feelings. It is not a finished process and probably never will be, but this very openness and lack of finality were sometimes interpreted as inconsistency. Then there is the difficulty of striking the right balance between guideline and prescription, maintaining the integrity and shape of the model while encouraging the adaptability needed for local ownership, which is critical for a successful project. We were accused of fuzziness if we tipped towards flexibility and of arrogance if we adhered to tighter criteria! Some nurses, regarding the criteria as more normative than descriptive, felt they were being judged and found wanting if their unit did not fulfil the criteria, even when the 'NDU model' was not appropriate to their circumstances or stage of development.

Despite the tension and frequent fears that we might be barking up the wrong tree, we pressed on to extrapolate assessment criteria from our conceptualisation of the NDU (Table 4.3). These criteria were to serve several purposes. The first was to help us and our

---

In assessing applications from individual units for grants to assist NDU development, the King's Fund Centre assessment team looked for evidence of work being undertaken on the following issues:

1. Commitment from health authority or equivalent body.
2. Statement of NDU purpose, aims and objectives.
3. Evaluation of nursing activities.
4. Investigation of a specific research topic.
5. Review of the unit's working practices.
6. Continuing education and development.
7. Autonomy of nursing practice.
8. Control of nursing budget.
9. Equal opportunities.
10. Sharing knowledge with a wider audience.
11. Liaison with other NDUs.

Table 4.3 Assessment criteria for NDUs (King's Fund 1988, see Appendix I)

advisers to assess the units which applied for inclusion in the NDU scheme. We had to choose the 'winners' according to our judgement of their readiness for change. We also wanted a framework to help us feed back ideas and impressions systematically to the staff.

The NDUs supported by the King's Fund Centre, we decided, would be those which aimed to meet the criteria used to assess the first round of applications. No unit could meet them all from the outset and many not even in the medium term. The criteria were not yardsticks to judge current performance, but pointers to the issues which we believed required close attention and we wanted to see how much thought had been given to them, even if the resources or ability to act on them were still lacking. We hoped the units would find them useful in formulating their goals and planning their strategies and that this would make the assessment process a learning experience for all involved, as much as a competition. They could be used as broad guidelines to help the units in their development – a kind of aide-mémoire of all the factors they needed to consider when embarking on change.

Although the criteria were not ranked in a strict order of priority, we decided that some were non-negotiable, based on the key features identified above. These included evidence that the unit's or team's philosophy valued and cherished all human beings, whether staff or patients; that belief in the value and potential of nursing was given; that the search for excellence was an unchanging aim; and that good human relationships were seen as the key to success. On the other hand, NDUs were not about prescription, regulation, one theory, one goal, one innovation, bricks and mortar or building from a blueprint. We were looking for teams of nurses who had ideas and enthusiasm for strengthening and building on their humanitarian values in the turbulent environment of contemporary health care. What, then, did we assess?

1. Commitment from the health authority or equivalent body

It is essential that the host organisation shows genuine commitment to the NDU project. Ideally, it should sign an agreement with the NDU specifying what support it is prepared to give, including financial and human resources. This encourages nurses and policy-makers to enter into dialogue, raises the nursing profile, increases understanding of nursing issues and makes the unit's future position more secure. (The survival prospects of the project beyond the initial three-year phase was an important consideration.)

2. Statement of NDU purpose, aims and objectives

An agreement specifying the purpose, aims and objectives of the NDU should be drawn up between practitioners, managers, other key staff and service users or their representatives. Details of the unit's philosophy and how it intends to meet these criteria should be included, with a timescale for achieving specified changes and for regular review.

3. Evaluation of nursing activities

The NDU should evaluate selected activities, including planned innovations, to determine their outcomes for patients. The yardsticks used should include effectiveness, efficiency, equity and acceptability. Other related considerations may include the effects on the working environment, staff recruitment and staff retention. Evaluation will involve using or refining existing qualitative and quantitative outcome measures or developing new ones.

4. Investigation of a specific nursing topic

Research-based nursing is a major NDU goal. Each unit investigates a specific nursing topic which is agreed by the staff to be of particular importance in patient care. The focus chosen varies according to local need and interest. Examples include the introduction of nursing beds, review of skill and staff mix, comparison of care delivery methods and the development of clinical nursing roles.

5. Review of the unit's working practices

Critical scrutiny of its own practice is a key activity. The unit should undertake continuing review and modification of its working practices, to take account of the results of evaluation within the NDU and elsewhere, using whatever method the staff agree is appropriate.

6. Continuing education and development

Change on the scale tackled by an NDU is impossible without a strong commitment to the continuing education and personal/professional development of all nursing staff. This should include individual development plans as well as group activities. Developing or strengthening links with appropriate institutions such as the local college of nursing, university nursing department or health authority in-service training unit is seen as an important support for this.

7. Autonomy of nursing practice

NDUs are expected to fight for the freedom for practitioners of nursing to control their own work, within a framework which is acceptable to patients, managers, doctors and other colleagues and which meets the requirements of other agencies such as Parliament, regulatory bodies and government health departments. This involves making nurses fully accountable for their practice and ensuring they have the authority to take decisions within the boundaries of their competence.

8. Control of nursing budget

Financial control is an important tool to gain autonomy for nursing practice. The NDU should aim to manage its own financial and other resources, working within an agreed budget. Control by clinical nurses of earmarked funds for staff development is highly desirable and essential if grants for this purpose have been given by external bodies such as the King's Fund or raised by the nurses themselves.

9. Equal opportunities

NDUs uphold the value of equity and respect for every individual person's rights. Equal opportunities policies should be developed and enforced for both staff and patients, covering such areas as discrimination on the grounds of race, gender, culture, religion and sexual orientation.

10. Sharing knowledge with a wider audience

NDUs are committed to the development of nursing as a whole, not only their own unit. The NDU should, in due course, disseminate its knowledge and experience to a wider multidisciplinary audience, using such means as study days, work placements, publications and consultancy.

11. Liaison with other NDUs

Doing innovative work can sometimes make staff feel lonely and isolated. Active liaison is sought with other NDUs or similar units, for mutual support and the exchange of information and experiences.

These criteria give a sketchy indication of the type of work which NDUs are tackling and how they are going about it. They do not, however, capture the variety and excitement of each unit's work, nor their unique flavour. Some of this can be found in the many accounts NDUs have already published in the nursing journals or presented at conferences (see the Select Bibliography); other accounts can be found elsewhere in this book. The four units which were chosen for development in the first round of the King's Fund programme illustrate the range of settings and activities undertaken:

- Brighton NDU is a 22-bed unit for the rehabilitation of elderly patients, based at Brighton General Hospital in Sussex. Care is organised through a primary nursing system. Among a number of projects carried out by staff, successes have included a project on reminiscence therapy and a multidisciplinary quality circle which led to improvements in patient safety. An action research project on the role of the nurse in rehabilitation is now under way.
- Camberwell NDU is a 17-bed female medical ward at Dulwich Hospital in south London. Staff are undertaking a major action research project on primary nursing and have developed ward-based individual performance review. Nursing work is audited using QUALPACS (Quality Patient Care Scale), a quality assurance tool developed in the USA.
- Southport NDU, at Southport General Infirmary in Lancashire, is a 26-bed ward for acute care of elderly patients. Staff are developing their own model of care and exploring how to make care more personal. A carers' panel has been formed to help identify the needs of patients and their relatives and introduce practical improvements.
- West Dorset NDU is a 24-bed female acute medical ward at the Weymouth and District Hospital in Dorset. It pioneered the use of Excelcare, a computerised system of nursing care planning and documentation. Primary nursing is being developed through an action research programme. Staff have joined self-awareness groups to help their personal growth and ability to cope with change.

Dilemmas, difficulties – and successes

Those brief descriptions of the four 'first-wave' NDUs supported by the King's Fund are the tip of the iceberg, as so much has happened in each unit over months and now years of collaborative work; it is hard to capture the true flavour of effort and achievement, of turmoil and insecurity. Perhaps the most significant changes in an NDU are the hardest to quantify, since they concern subtle but crucial shifts in people's attitudes and assumptions – shifts that create the climate in which innovations of all kinds can flourish. The business of an NDU is to improve patient care, not merely by introducing one specific innovation, but by changing its culture to one where innovation is a continuing process. Gradually and cumulatively, it also helps to transform the overall culture of nursing and health care.

Changing human attitudes and behaviour is the most complex of all activities and establishing an NDU on a secure foundation is a complex process. Lasting success depends on a variety of factors ranging from good leadership to grass-roots support. It is a slow and sometimes painful business, requiring a great deal of energy and commitment from people who are often already overloaded with the needs and demands of others, whether patients or colleagues. It is difficult to put into practice in everyday life the values of the NDU movement, with its emphasis on equity and respect for self and others.

The selection process outlined above aimed to ensure that the units with which our Nursing Developments Programme worked were ripe for change and able to cope with these challenges: we wanted to back winners. This pragmatism was necessary in view of our limited development resources, but it was also clear from experience that changing nursing, even in the most supportive and prosperous environments, is an uphill struggle – no one would have an easy ride in these supposedly elite units. Furthermore, the success of the winners would blaze the trail for others.

Our strategic decision to back potential winners was often criticised. Many nurses felt uncomfortable with the notion of a centre of excellence even though they could see that, rationally speaking, such centres were essential for progress. While NDUs do not claim the 'centre of excellence' label for themselves and even tend to underplay their achievements, other nurses sometimes put them on a pedestal in order to knock them down. Typically, I heard a nurse after a visit to Tameside NDU commenting with great relish that her ward back home did things much better and NDUs obviously weren't what they were cracked up to be! Yet the Tameside staff had taken great pains to encourage discussion of what they had done and often said they did not have all the answers.

Experiences such as the closure of the Oxford NDU (Salvage 1989) have led people to question the wisdom of establishing units to become centres of excellence – raising heads above the parapet seems too dangerous. Despite the risks, we felt that the time was right for nursing to come out of its shell and to be more open and assertive about its dreams and its achievements. In the competitive environment of health care today, those who are unwilling to wave their own flag find themselves forgotten, powerless and penniless, a fact of life we have to acknowledge, however much we may deplore it. By adopting a relatively high profile, a nursing flagship such as an NDU could be a vital force in raising morale and demonstrating the art of the possible.

As the NDUs entered the public eye through journal articles and conferences, the double-edged effects of fame became apparent. Efforts to keep the NDUs as 'protected environments' where the staff could work undisturbed were sometimes hard to sustain. Other nurses were keen to visit the unit and of course the staff were keen to receive them, to exchange ideas and to bask in a little well-earned glory. However, living in a goldfish bowl has its problems and after a while the units started to organise open days and other means of controlling the flow of onlookers. Linked with this was the pressure of other people's expectations; the units' achievements were not always dramatic and the pace of change is never even, yet people – visitors, general managers, doctors – seemed to expect miracles overnight. Since nurses already tend to have impossibly high expectations of themselves, reinforced by the traditional professional culture (Hingley and Cooper 1986), this provided great opportunities for gloom and self-flagellation.

The charge that NDUs are elitist, even if it is not justified, should be taken seriously for what it reveals about nurses' individual and collective psychology. Low self-esteem and lack of confidence, instilled in women from an early age, are reinforced by socialisation as a nurse and help create deep-seated insecurity in the profession. Putting others down is a familiar coping mechanism and NDUs have had to deal with surprising hostility from nursing colleagues – as though even daring to articulate the aim of excellence is unacceptable. This phenomenon was clearly at work in the demise of Oxford NDU, where many nurses working in the same hospital ignored or even undermined the unit's work; their insecurity also manifested itself in a refusal to tolerate differences.

Conflict was not only apparent between the units and other nurses. As the work progressed we were surprised by how much conflict surfaced within the unit teams and between our team and the units, as well as within our own team. With hindsight it is not surprising, given the difficulty of the work, the strong personalities involved and the high levels of uncertainty, but at the time it seemed shocking that nurses with so many shared aspirations should be in conflict with each other. Finding good ways to handle conflict was a key to success, because otherwise, creative work was very difficult. This was all the harder because conflict tended to be hidden or unacknowledged in the units.

Experiencing conflict within our own team, which was sometimes the result of containing or being infected by the units' tensions, was distressing but we usually managed to face up to it, having asked expert consultants at the outset to help us develop processes for handling it in an empowering way. Knowing how difficult we found this, even in our own supportive and stable team, we could understand how hard it was for the NDUs, with all the added pressures they faced. They usually resisted our attempts to bring into the open the fears and insecurities which we as outsiders thought were the source of many of their internal tensions, presumably for fear that open disagreement would blow their team apart – so they would deny there was a problem. They were also reluctant to be open about their disagreements with us, even when the atmosphere could be cut with a knife. Obviously the King's Fund power and money were a factor, for even though we encouraged open debate and tried to avoid hidden agendas, the units probably feared that open disagreement would jeopardise the relationship and even the funding.

Jealousy and covert hostility appear to arise in some form in each NDU, but they do not invalidate the NDU strategy. We learned from the Oxford experience by attempting to minimise the factors which contributed to its closure, as demonstrated in the assessment criteria. Moreover, the forces of resistance are to be found in every change process – with skilful handling they can be transformed into creative energy. The same tensions and emotions also exist inside each one of us and in every professional team: the point is to learn how to deal with them well, rather than to deny or avoid them.

Another aspect of the elitism charge which frequently arises is that of fairness. Shouldn't everyone have a share of the NDU goodies? Yet nursing development resources are usually meagre and when spread too thinly they make no impact. Too many nurses are burning themselves out in posts where they are expected to develop nursing practice in an entire hospital – single-handed. On the other hand, there is evidence that with the right motivation and support, nurses are adept at securing resources and often just need a nudge (praise and recognition and a small grant) to help them on their way.

Our strategic choices were also directed by an underlying theory of change. This was eclectic but drew heavily on previous clinical nursing 'experiments', primarily Burford, Oxford and Tameside NDUs, which in turn had been inspired by Ottaway (1976), among others. Ottaway's concept of the pilot site was crucial: a selected setting which introduces and internalises new norms and eventually helps them to spread across the whole organisation. As the change takes root, other units may challenge the pilot site's change agent role and indeed overtake it as a powerhouse of innovation; the inevitable competitive edge is therefore a source of creativity and no one can rest on their laurels. Interlinked factors include the need for change to be perceived, owned and driven by the participants themselves, as discussed earlier.

Robustness of the model

These tricky issues and the many others which form the meat and drink of development work are helping to shape and refine the model of the NDU. It is relatively simple to design such a model on paper, but the project has always been rooted in experience as well as vision, so the refinement process is a constant interplay between learning from experience, new theory and pragmatism. Model as a term feels too restrictive for what we are doing and lends itself too easily to mechanistic interpretations or assumptions about replicability which are inappropriate to social institutions such as health services. Nevertheless there are broad criteria, as outlined earlier, which can be applied to determine whether a unit is functioning as an NDU on the lines advocated by the King's Fund Centre. It is also important to tackle head-on the questions about robustness and transferability, since health services will only invest in NDUs if they are persuaded that real benefits will ensue.

The NDU model has already proved its success in some respects and in some settings. As with all such projects it is impossible to prove that it can work for all time and in all places, since success depends on many variables. What sample of successful NDUs would be taken as sufficient proof and what criteria constitute success? Previous research studies and the current evaluation work provide some pointers, while the complexities of replicability are extensively discussed in the social science literature. Bachrach, in a fascinating discussion of demonstration projects for mentally ill people in the USA, warns of the need 'to shift from the habit of looking to demonstration projects as solutions, to integrating what we learn from them into the fabric of service planning' (Bachrach 1988). The experimental/model programmes she describes could not be copied or generalised to other settings beyond certain 'simple commonalities', such as strong leadership and individualised care planning. 'These commonalities are so simple that they may prove to be a disappointment to those people who look to demonstration projects to provide them with sophisticated or "sexy" solutions for their own problems,' she notes. We have the same feelings about our NDU commonalities or 'key features' identified above; yet the simplest and most obvious points are often the hardest to achieve.

Bachrach gives several reasons why projects could not be reproduced elsewhere beyond those commonalities. Every project has its own cultural context and milieu; it is hard to know what makes a successful project work; the projects attract exceptional staff and often have extra resources or other benefits. Moreover, a project may be very successful in its own right but have no impact, or perhaps even a negative one, on other people in need. Successful projects tell us only that demonstration projects work and cloning is not their reason for existence.

A further factor in assessing the 'success' of an NDU is the broader context of nursing development. The need for and nature of clinical practice development is only just beginning to be recognised, alongside an awareness that many different approaches to development are needed – despite the temptation to believe in panaceas. NDUs as an unsupported, isolated development cannot change the face of nursing: they are just one promising option in a range of possibilities.

Nevertheless, widespread and long-term practice development is unlikely to occur in a hospital or community unit which lacks a workplace-based focus for such activities. Unless the host organisation is exceptionally wealthy, uncomfortable choices have to be made about where limited resources for practice development should be allocated. The controversial question of NDU size (one ward, two wards, several, a whole hospital? A community team or an entire neighbourhood?) is thus determined by pragmatism as well as change theory. The appropriateness of the NDU model to different settings is also problematic; to date, the majority have specialised in hospital care of the elderly, though there are thriving NDUs in intensive care, acute surgery and elsewhere. The principles or commonalities are applicable to any setting, though feasibility also depends on factors such as medical power, which is related to speciality. Another question is the applicability of the model to non-hospital settings, midwifery, care settings which involve large groups of staff working in a single integrated unit and genuinely multidisciplinary teams.

The King's Fund role

One source of our dilemmas was also a source of strength – perhaps like all dilemmas, as growth comes in the attempt to resolve them. The issue of ownership of the NDU model has already been touched on, but mainly in terms of the need for staff within NDUs to be the owners and drivers of the change. However, the issue of ownership was also complicated at times in relation to the King's Fund. On the one hand, it was always clear that the NDUs with whom we worked in partnership were the owners of their projects; however closely involved our Nursing Developments Team became, we would never be insiders. On the other hand, we invested a great deal in the units – commitment, support, advice, energy and money. As Gillian Black relates more fully in Chapter 7, we tried many means of strengthening the partnership, including agreeing a contract with each NDU which clarified both sides' expectations and obligations.

Despite the strength of the partnerships, issues inevitably arose where agreement was difficult and disputes over ownership then came to the fore. The units were doing their own work in their own way and, as they sometimes pointed out, they would have done so with or without us. Yet from our perspective they had agreed to join a collaborative project based on specific principles. If we feared that a particular NDU's course of action would compromise the 'model', it was hard to know how far we should insist on compliance if persuasion failed. We felt a dissonance between our belief that the NDUs should own their project and our need to adhere to our programme's goals, for the sake of future as well as current developments. Fortunately, a compromise could usually be found and the issue did not often surface overtly, but when it did it was extremely stressful all round.

Such dilemmas reminded us that the innovative aspects of the NDU programme were not confined to the units themselves. The nature of the partnership between the NDUs and the King's Fund was also breaking new ground in nursing. Our team had much to offer to the units, but that did not include experience of this type of partnership, where we were not simply grant-givers but also working partners. We shared the units' feeling that they often had to make it up as they went along. The uncertainty this created in our own team could be hard to cope with, but it was also a strength, since we were not simply advising the NDUs from a theoretical standpoint, but experiencing for ourselves similar processes of change and growth.

Laying bare our experience of these difficult processes was one way of acting as a resource for the NDUs – providing technical advice, ideas and information but also emotional support. We encouraged networking between the units and organised regular events to bring everyone together, although we were often disappointed that the discussions were not very open: the latent rivalry between the units was surprisingly high and people were reluctant to be honest about difficulties we knew they were experiencing. This seemed to spring from the lack of confidence discussed earlier and the linked fear of appearing incompetent. The constructive critique and open scrutiny to which everyone paid lip-service usually proved in practice to be forced on the units by us.

The fact that we were not simply grant-givers should not obscure the important though by no means dominant role of money in the relationship between the NDUs and the Fund. Even though the grants were no more than £30 000 a year for the four units, and as low as £1000 for other NDUs, the need to develop mechanisms to ensure the money was spent as earmarked helped us both to protect the integrity of the projects in cash-starved health authorities and to influence the overall financial status of the units.

The backing of an authoritative, independent, national organisation brought considerable benefits to the NDUs. Many of the doctors and probably all the general managers involved knew of the Fund and respected it; with the general managers in particular this gave us an important entry point and reassured them of our commitment to health service development in general rather than narrow professional concerns. This enabled us to play a brokerage role if need be, mediating between the needs of the NDU and the general managers when these diverged, especially in the units' steering groups. The legitimation conferred by King's Fund backing also gave the NDUs added prestige and credibility in their host organisations and brought hitherto unacknowledged achievements to the attention of senior people. Our role as 'product champion' of NDUs also allowed us to highlight their progress and to lobby for nursing development resources, not only within the nursing profession nationally but also in circles normally closed to clinical nurses. Our finest hour in that respect was a dinner hosted by the

Fund and attended by the Secretary of State for Health, the chief executive of the NHS and other luminaries of the health policy and management scene, who rubbed shoulders with NDU clinical leaders. Some of the dignitaries later commented that they had never before appreciated the depth of talent and commitment among clinical nurses, while the nurses had an unprecedented opportunity to put their case to key decision-makers. In fact, we were demonstrating in action one of the Fund's strongest assets: the ability and authority to make the strategic link between policy-making and practice.

Conclusion

In an account such as this it is perhaps easier to focus on the difficulties than the good times, especially as the fruits of development work are often slow to ripen. It should be clear that there are no right answers – but perhaps plenty of wrong ones! – in work of this kind, although some approaches seem to work much better than others. Looking back, now that I am no longer directly involved in the NDU programme, my impressions are overwhelmingly positive. Working with people of such energy and commitment in the NDUs and in my team, seeing their efforts gradually flowering, seeing them grow as people and knowing that my own development advanced in leaps and bounds – these are experiences all too rare in our working lives. It was a privilege to be a part of that and now to continue the learning and the growth in the broader European setting of my current work with the World Health Organization. Whatever the final place of NDUs in the health care system – and I am sure they will be around for some time to come – the path we travelled together is a rewarding one.

References

Bachrach L (1988) *Demonstration Projects for Chronic Mental Patients: Advantages and Pitfalls*. Unpublished paper. For further discussion see Bachrach L (1988) On exporting and importing model programs. *Hospital and Community Psychiatry* **39**(12): 1257–1258.

Beardshaw V and Robinson R (1990) *New for Old? Prospects for Nursing in the 1990s*. King's Fund Institute Research Report No. 8. London: King's Fund.

Hingley P and Cooper C (1986) *Stress and the Nurse Manager*. Chichester: John Wiley and Sons.

Ottaway R (1976) A change strategy to implement new norms, new styles and new environments in the work organisation. *Personnel Review* 5(1): 13–15.

Salvage J (1989) Setback for nursing. *Nursing Times*, 85(11): 19.

Salvage J (1992) The New Nursing: Empowering Patients or Empowering Nurses? In J Robinson, A Gray and R Elkan (eds) *Policy Issues in Nursing*. Milton Keynes: Open University Press.

Stocking B (1985) *Initiative and Inertia: Case Studies in the NHS*. London: Nuffield Provincial Hospitals Trust.

Towell D and Harries C (eds) (1979) *Innovation in Patient Care*. London: Croom Helm.

Wright S (1989) Defining the nursing development unit. *Nursing Standard* 4(7): 29-31.

CHAPTER 5

Managing the Changes

Jane Salvage

In the first four chapters of this book we have concentrated on describing the background to the NDU initiative and explaining its main theoretical underpinnings. Now we can turn to the more practical question of how to get an NDU off the ground and how to keep it going – in other words, how to manage the change. Some of the ideas on managing change which emerged from our experience of nursing practice development have been described at greater length by Wright (1989).

It has already been emphasised that each NDU has its own unique features, circumstances and personalities and that this rich diversity is to be welcomed. This diversity is also illustrated in the many different ways in which the units have started up, each reflecting its own local environment. Even the broad assertion that an NDU has to adopt a 'bottom-up' approach – created and inspired by nurses at the grass roots – appears inadequate when we look at the history of the units.

The four pilot NDUs in the King's Fund scheme all had support in their early days from the top as well as the bottom, although to different degrees. The programme initially placed greater emphasis on the bottom-up approach, mainly because we felt more comfortable with the human values it implies, but also because we thought success was more likely this way and we needed to pick winners in the programme's vulnerable early stages. Bottom-up support from the outset will take the unit a long way. And as it makes progress, it is likely to attract some interest from the top. It is a hard task, although not an impossible one, to use a top-down approach when no one at the bottom seems interested, as all managers know. The gap between top and bottom has to be narrowed in any successful project and a symbiosis of both approaches is better than dogmatic adherence to one or the other.

An NDU can, in fact, be born of the enthusiasm of any group of nurses. Usually that initial energy comes from clinical staff, but it can also come from nurse managers, educationalists, researchers and general managers; there were examples of each type in the King's Fund NDU network. My first contact with one of the four pilot NDUs came from a phone call from a management consultant, not a nurse, working temporarily in a regional health authority. He then visited me at the King's Fund Centre, accompanied by a district general manager and a chief nursing officer. The three men in their business suits crammed into my tiny office to tell me about their great dedication to clinical nursing and their plans for nursing development in the district. Somewhat sceptical, I lectured them on the importance of the project being led and owned by clinical nurses rather than by senior managers, showed them the door and never thought I would see them again. They persisted and managed to find a group of clinical nurses keen to run with the idea: the NDU they helped to establish has done marvellous work!

The starting point for the NDU, then, will vary from place to place and each has its pros and cons. Sometimes, though not inevitably, a strong lead from management may mean disempowerment of clinical staff, an educational emphasis may alienate some service staff, and so on; furthermore, each group will have its own legitimate agenda which will not be quite the same as everyone else's. In any case, the starting point cannot be prescribed, as it will depend on the focus of energy and desire for change and the ability to act on it. Some health authorities are experimenting with ways of identifying those high-energy spots by holding an open competition in which they ask teams of nurses to nominate themselves for NDU status by submitting proposals for assessment by their peers and managers. This helps to minimise the charges of favouritism or hidden agendas which inevitably arise when a unit is simply selected by managers and helps them to formulate a phased development plan for an entire service or management unit. The competition, carefully conducted, can also be a useful spur to clinical teams to stimulate interest in new ideas and to clarify their goals.

Doing your homework

The next steps to be taken in the development process are broadly similar in principle whatever the starting point for the NDU. These will be the main focus of this chapter. It will be assumed here that you, the reader, are a member of a community or ward nursing team, although the material is also relevant to managers, teachers and researchers. It will also be assumed that you are interested in your unit becoming an NDU and that you have done your homework – that you are already familiar with the basic concepts and the literature. (See the Select Bibliography at the end of this book) This may seem obvious, but it is surprising how many people either want to become an NDU or else are hostile to the idea without actually knowing what an NDU is or studying the literature.

Before going any further it may be worthwhile thinking through, or even better talking through with a colleague, why you want to have an NDU. It is only one of many ways of tackling nursing development and perhaps a different strategy would be more suitable in your circumstances. What are your goals and what do you want to change? What is the best way to get there? The process of development, while exhilarating, is also arduous. You will need all the help you can get, so your choice of strategy – finding the best means to reach your ends – is critical.

Some of this initial thinking and, of course, the background reading can be done on your own, but it is better done as a team. If you are unsure how your colleagues feel about making changes in the team's work, you can organise an informal discussion among the keen ones, those who will drive the changes. This is the beginning of the change cycle, a process that fosters successful growth whether you are trying to make changes in a small team, a big hospital or a commercial company.

The change cycle is depicted in Figure 5.1. It is similar to the formulation found in many management textbooks, but this version is the work of management consultant Robin Coates. As this figure shows, the cyclical, self-renewing nature of the process is crucial: it is not a series of steps to be taken once only, but is a continuing process of change and review. Real life is not systematic like a diagram – each activity influences and interacts with the other activities and not necessarily in the order shown. However, clarifying the steps and making sure attention is paid to each one helps us to make sense of the muddle of real life and to start to shape it as we want it.

Another perspective underpinning the cycle is the idea that 'success' is in many ways a journey rather than a destination. By the time the project reaches the goal originally planned, it is likely to have undergone so many changes that it may be barely recognisable; the bigger the project, the more likely this is. This is not a sign of failure, but reflects the reality of human endeavour, learning, changing and adapting as we go along. This highlights the importance of the process itself. The journey is as important as the end-point and the way we go about change may be as important as the change itself – as well as having a huge influence on the outcome.

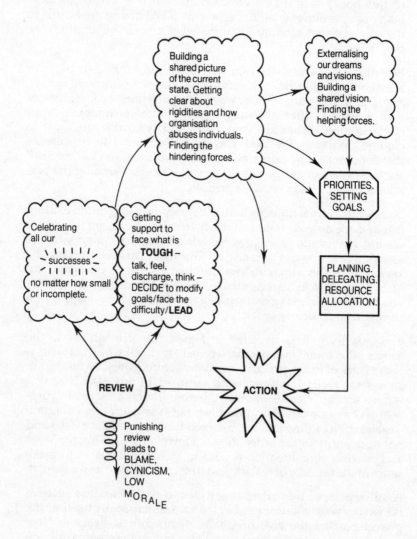

Figure 5.1 The change cycle in organisations/teams

The change cycle and NDUs

How, then, can the change cycle help NDU development? Its main steps, together with the key NDU features and assessment criteria outlined in Chapter 4, provide a series of milestones or building blocks for the project, a kind of checklist for action or discussion. Not all the steps may always be necessary, but in our experience, omitting or skipping any of them leads to trouble later on. Careful preparation and a systematic approach will not solve all the problems, but will certainly help you to tackle them more effectively and to predict – and therefore pre-empt – some of them.

1. Assessing the current situation

The desire to change often originates in dissatisfaction with the current situation. Talk to any nurse about her work and usually you will hear a litany of complaints and anxieties: surveys show that most nurses are unhappy about the quality of patient care and the lack of value placed on nursing itself and doubtful of their own capabilities. The challenge is to refocus the energy we put into complaining or feeling inadequate into a positive force for change – making canteen grumbles the subject of team meetings and turning individual hopelessness into shared commitment. Encourage your team to build a collective picture of the current state. People will be only too keen to talk about how they think the organisation – the boss, the doctors, management or just 'them' – prevents them from doing what they want, how it abuses them and how it obstructs change. Change agents, perhaps being optimists by nature, are often impatient with such talk, but it is a key starting point, a way of clearing the ground. As well as discharging negative feelings, the analysis it contains will be invaluable in developing strategies and tactics.

2. Building a shared vision

Once people have had a chance to express their feelings about the current situation and pinpoint some of the forces which they think will hinder change, they may be ready to build a vision of how they would like their work and their lives to be. These dreams and visions are not idle fantasies or useless philosophy, as they are sometimes labelled by action-oriented people, but essential catalysts for change. Unfortunately, most of us are so used to negative thinking that it is hard to get back in touch with our most deeply held values and aspirations. We are embarrassed if we sound idealistic and we censor our dreams before we have barely acknowledged them to ourselves, let alone externalised them. People are also cynical about 'visions' and 'missions' because of the current fashion among many organisations to produce high-sounding statements without consultation that belie the everyday reality of the organisation's aims and working practices.

Helping people to express their dreams and visions can therefore be difficult, but it is not impossible. Many, if not most, nurses enter the profession with high ideals and positive visions of how they want to help others. Those ideals may have become bruised and battered on the way, but they probably still exist, based on the person's individual value system. For real teamwork those value systems need to be discussed and the shared values identified. These can then be formulated into a written or pictorial statement if desired, as a touchstone of what is important – although the statement is not in itself the goal of vision-building.

The interest in primary nursing has provided some good examples of how nurses can develop shared visions. The stimulus has come from valuing the importance of respect for each patient or client as an individual. From this basic value, nurses have developed a vision of how it can underpin their practice – by thinking about what perfect patient care might look and feel like and then working out how to make that a reality. Whether this is called a philosophy, an ethic or a mission, it reflects the importance of connecting with people's individual aspirations and beliefs, identifying the common ground and fusing individual values into a shared vision with which the whole team feels comfortable. During this process the team is also likely to identify forces which will help it to achieve its goals.

3. Setting goals

Now your team is ready to convert its vision into reality. This is best tackled by formulating goals or objectives based on the different aspects of the vision. For example, the vision of patient-centred care could partly be achieved through the goal of introducing a new system of care management. An important way of agreeing the goals is to have brainstorming sessions with the team – bringing up any and every idea however crazy it seems, then using a democratic process to reach consensus on which goals should be the priority.

The first NDU work plans we saw were nearly always unrealistic because they were so long and ambitious. Nurses often find it difficult to choose priorities. Our professional socialisation, combined with the pressures of the organisation, tells us that we should meet every need and never say no. However, it is impossible to meet every need. By spreading ourselves too thinly and trying to do everything we work less effectively and put ourselves under more stress than if we had a clear focus in view. Setting unrealistic goals demotivates people when they fail to reach them and reinforces their feelings of failure. Achieving a target within a manageable plan, on the other hand, gives confidence and a sense of direction.

4. Planning

Once the priority goals are agreed they should be sorted into a work plan. Each team member should have the sense that this plan belongs to them and has their commitment, so everyone should be involved in agreeing the plan – perhaps by drawing up a draft together, delegating a group member to produce a more polished version and then reviewing it. Each goal needs to be considered in detail, deciding what needs to be done to achieve it: what the helping forces will be and how they can be harnessed; what the hindering forces will be and how they can be reduced; who will be responsible for each component task, including the establishment of steering groups and work groups; where the human and financial resources will come from; and the timescale. This plan then serves as the referral point, the basis of review and the guide to action. It will usually be modified in the light of experience, but changes should be made openly in full discussion with the team.

5. Action

The action plan drawn up by the team provides the main reference point for its work. In the busy world of the health service, action is the dominant feature of every nurse's working life, and most nurses are very good at being, or at least appearing, active. In the bad old days, the demand to 'look busy' meant that non-physical forms of activity, such as sitting by a distressed person, were culturally unacceptable. Although traces of that attitude still persist, nursing has now developed a more sophisticated interpretation of action which values emotional and intellectual as well as physical work and which emphasises the importance of results as a guide to setting priorities. We are less prone to do things for the sake of ticking them off a list or because they are routine and more likely to consider first whether the activity is actually necessary.

Nevertheless, one of the biggest difficulties experienced by NDUs is creating enough space for reflection and learning, psychologically as well as in time and space, and in the daily context of the job as well as on more formal occasions such as seminars and study days. Symbolically, the lack of comfortable meeting rooms for staff near the work area shows the low priority given to such activity in the NHS. Everyone needs continual reassurance that talking to each other, discussing issues during work time, reading or simply taking a few minutes for silence and peace in the middle of a frantic day is as legitimate and important as the endless rushing around.

Another issue likely to arise in the 'action' phase of the change cycle is the probability that things will not go quite as planned. However systematic and thorough the planning has been, and however well it is supported by staff and patients, life has a way of producing the unforeseen. Provided time is made available to recognise what is happening and to consider the implications, the unpredictable can be a source of creativity as the person or the team uses its resources to adapt to the new situation and to see what possibilities it holds, rather than sticking dogmatically to the workplan or using inappropriate coping mechanisms learned elsewhere as survival strategies.

6. Review

The importance of review will already be apparent from the comments above. The technical aspects of evaluation, a systematic and scientific form of review, are discussed by Rebecca Malby in Chapter 9. Here my emphasis is on the need for everyone involved in change to have frequent opportunities, as individuals and as teams, to review what they are doing and what they think and feel about it. One important form of review is to celebrate our successes, no matter how small or incomplete; everyone appreciates recognition and praise and a team celebration of a milestone reached provides more motivation to tackle the next stage. Sometimes it can be a simple matter of a pat on the back; at other times the success may merit a meal out for the whole team or a professional treat such as buying new books for the unit.

Review can also mean getting support to face what is tough – talking, feeling, expressing and discharging emotions and thinking may be necessary before enough clarity can be found to help decide how to modify goals or behaviours, make new plans, face the difficulty and exercise leadership. Reviews of successes and difficulties can range from a 10-minute chat between two people to a full-scale formal team meeting, depending on what needs reviewing and what approach is best. Yet although there are no set rules, the need for frequent review cannot be avoided and it will in fact be welcomed once people learn how helpful it can be. It gradually becomes inherent in the work, a part of the continuing cycle of change rather than a single end-stage, and it will often lead to further adaptation and change.

Many people have a problem with reviewing because most of us still expect it to involve an assessment of us, in which we will be found wanting. Educational systems which rely primarily on examinations, tests and grades – where we are always judged not in our own right but in competition with others – cause deep-rooted harm by linking all subsequent types of evaluation with expectations of punishment and reward. Those who do well are always fearful of 'failing' next time, while those who 'fail' lose self-confidence and become dispirited. The kinds of review used in nursing must avoid any association with punishment, which leads to guilt, blame and cynicism. Instead, they should emphasise review as a form of celebration and learning, whose purpose is to help us and to liberate our creativity.

Other keys to success

In Chapter 2 Steve Wright described how change in NDUs is supported by planned programmes of personal and professional development. These provide the ballast or scaffolding for the change cycle activities outlined above. This emphasis on development is, of course, a feature not only of NDUs but of many successful organisations, be they humanitarian or commercial. Another way of conceptualising it is shown in Figure 5.2 below in which three overlapping circles represent the three main areas of activity of the ideal organisation: strategy, implementation and improvement. Each is vital to success and each needs to be given its fair share of attention; each is interlinked with the other two.

Many organisations do not maintain a good balance between the three areas, however. Most divide their staff into dysfunctional hierarchies in which a few powerful people do strategic work and the rest carry out the plans – in theory, at least! – with only a small, marginalised department to lead on development and training, and limited communication between the three areas. This leads to the separation of components that should be closely interlinked: thinking and action, data and perceptions, policy and operation, planning and implementation, experts and workers. Evidence shows that close integration of strategy and operations, with opportunities for all staff to undertake both types of work, is highly effective – especially when development receives much attention and therefore enhances people's capacities in the other two areas.

The NHS is currently an organisation in which the three circles hardly overlap and are disproportionately sized. Strategic planning is improving (and more closely tied to health outcomes), but it is poorly reflected in operational activity, which still drives the organisation, while development is neglected. Yet experience in NDUs shows that it is possible to work in a different way despite the shortcomings of the dominant culture. When NDUs have problems, the power of that dominant culture often seems to block change; but where due attention is paid to the work of development and improvement, staff and service users are empowered to take responsibility for change and to drive it through. Investment in development is not a frill or an airy-fairy notion, but an essential tool for progress.

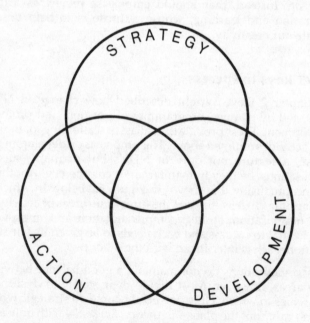

Figure 5.2 The ideal organisation

When we talk about development with our colleagues, someone inevitably comments, 'We'd like to do it, but we can't afford it.' Winning friends, influencing people and raising money are inevitable, practical but sometimes less welcome activities associated with an NDU. They are all made easier by using a change process such as that outlined above, because the clearer and more systematic the work programme and the sharper the goals and focus, the easier it is to explain it to others and gain their support. NDU leaders have learned to become salespeople and entrepreneurs, fundraisers and propagandists – perhaps not quite what they envisaged for their nursing career, but invaluable for their units! What kind of activities are they now undertaking?

Writing reports and proposals

NDUs and other development projects increasingly rely on external funding, from local charities for example, or from national grant-giving bodies. Even for internal funding, resources are no longer allocated automatically but must be competed for. A good case must be made for any bid, almost always in the form of a written report or proposal outlining the aims of the project, the expected outcomes, the action plan, the form of evaluation to be carried out and the estimated cost. Anyone who has vetted proposals knows how dreary they can be and how exciting it is to read a stimulating, persuasive and well-presented document. Sometimes the written document must be backed up by a verbal presentation and similar skills are needed when the time comes to report to the health authority, trust or project steering group. Guidance and courses on these 'non-nursing' activities are widely available (see, for example, Tierney 1989) and are increasingly regarded as core skills for the senior nurse.

Securing funding

NDUs have begun to secure funds from surprising as well as obvious sources by using their planning and presentation skills and their sheer ingenuity. Some, for example, encourage patients who offer boxes of chocolates to contribute instead to a development fund (NDUs are even good for your waistline). Such funds, held by the unit leader, can provide bursaries to unit staff, allocated by the staff themselves. They can also be a source of income generation by providing core funding for study days and publications. Some NDUs have built partnerships with local charities and self-help groups, which may provide assistance or help to raise funds. Some have been surprised by what they have managed to raise once they are clear about their objectives and have used local community networks and the media to publicise their aspirations and achievements.

Winning friends and influencing people

Preparing successful proposals and securing funding are part of the process of winning friends and influencing people. Again, such skills may seem alien to today's nurse, but the profession's lack of them in the past has been one of the causes – albeit not the main one – of its invisibility. Winning support and resources means making visible the work of nursing, especially its active contribution to health, replacing the traditional passive image of hand-holding and fevered brow-soothing. In the early stages of the change cycle, analysing the helping and hindering forces will suggest who needs to be persuaded, cajoled, won over, neutralised or otherwise enlisted to the cause of the fledgling NDU, whether it is a sceptical chief executive, an indifferent senior nurse or an enthusiastic doctor. Plans of campaign can then be devised to make sure that responsibilities for this lobbying are clearly allocated, deadlines set and activities reviewed.

Communication

This is another key to success. Free, frequent and open communication within the NDU is essential to create the trusting atmosphere and supportive climate in which creativity can flourish. This climate will then positively influence those who come into contact with the NDU, whether as patients, carers, staff or managers. A similar free flow of communication is also vital with all those outside the unit who matter to its functioning and future, from the catering manager to the chief consultant.

Knowing what and when to communicate is not always easy; some units have found themselves wilting in the hothouse glare of new and sometimes unwelcome publicity. Nursing developments start life as fragile plants and the temperature in the NDU greenhouse needs to be monitored carefully. Even visits by other nurses, fun and flattering though they may be at first, can become a chore. Some NDUs control the flow by admitting professional visitors on set days (and charging a fee to raise money). Deciding when and what to publish in the professional press is also problematic. Although managers, health authorities and the Department of Health may unrealistically demand instant success, innovations should be firmly rooted before being exposed to outside scrutiny, especially as seeming to claim too much too soon can lead to disenchantment among staff and attract hostility from others.

The ripple effect

However systematically and thoughtfully you approach it, developing nursing in an NDU is always challenging, sometimes frustrating and frequently unpredictable. At the centre of it all there is you, the individual nurse, intermittently prone to feelings of uncertainty and ill-equipped for such an adventurous project. So remember to enjoy your successes. When the going gets tough, you can still be a positive influence; we all make a difference. What follows is an inspiring reminder from *The Tao of Leadership* (Heider 1985):

Do you want to be a positive influence in the world? First, get your own life in order. Ground yourself in the single principle so that your behaviour is wholesome and effective. If you do that, you will earn respect and be a powerful influence.

Your behaviour influences others through a ripple effect. A ripple effect works because everyone influences everyone else. Powerful people are powerful influences.

If your life works, you influence your family.

If your family works, your family influences the community.
If your community works, your community influences the nation.
If your nation works, your nation influences the world.
If your world works, the ripple effect spreads throughout the cosmos.
Remember that your influence begins with you and ripples outward. So be sure that your influence is both potent and wholesome.
How do I know that this works?
All growth spreads outward from a fertile and potent nucleus.
You are a nucleus.

References

Heider J (1985) *The Tao of Leadership: Lao Tzu's 'Tao Te Ching' adapted for a New Age*. Atlanta, Ga: Humanics New Age.
Tierney A (1989) Grantsmanship: Resources for nursing research. *Senior Nurse* 9(2): 9.
Wright S (1989) *Changing Nursing Practice*. London: Edward Arnold.

CHAPTER 6

Developing Nurses – some internal strategies

Gillian Black

I joined the King's Fund Centre Nursing Developments Programme as a project worker in July 1989, just as the first four King's Fund Centre NDUs were being selected. My remit was to work with the four selected units in Brighton, Camberwell, Southport and West Dorset over a three-year period as they implemented their plans for developing nursing practice. As the King's Fund Centre project progressed I also gave some support to other units which joined the NDU network. It is from the collaboration with these units that I have drawn examples to illustrate this chapter and the next.

Why develop nurses?

It will have become apparent in previous chapters that the NDU concept is underpinned by a philosophy which generally takes an optimistic view of human nature and values people's creative and dynamic abilities, including working innovatively in groups. If that is the case, fostering that creativity will lead to the development of nursing practice. It was also apparent both from the experiences of other nurses who had developed nursing practice prior to the King's Fund Centre project and from our experiences as the project progressed that there were other compelling but related reasons for developing nurses.

Changes in nursing practice, the prime purpose of an NDU, inevitably require new knowledge and skills and often new attitudes as well. These need to be established at a variety of levels. A change in practice will probably require a nurse to develop new clinical skills and to acquire more knowledge. In order to effect that change she may equally be required to develop skills in 'selling' the change to the organisation, negotiating with management and

89

acquiring knowledge about financial bidding within her provider unit.

Sometimes it is also necessary to be aware of and overcome defensive behaviours unconsciously learned to protect ourselves or to protect others. It is helpful to remember that much of our training until recently was aimed at protecting patients who were largely being nursed by an unqualified workforce; dire warnings left many nurses feeling that nothing should ever go wrong and they consequently adopted a very controlling attitude to their work and to others. A major organisational weakness became internalised in us as individuals.

The overall project gave the Nursing Developments Programme the chance to explore three fundamental areas in the development of nurses. These were:

- The development of new roles
- New empowering relationships between nurses and patients and among nurses
- New strategies for personal and professional development

All three areas influence one another; while each unit approached the subject of staff development very differently, a constant transformation of approaches was under way: new roles leading to different strategies for personal and professional development, and new relationships between patients and nurses leading to nurses taking on different roles in the nursing team.

New roles

The project supported new development posts in each NDU to help bring about change in practice. In many respects these new posts had something in common with my post as project worker. There were misconceptions about the posts which the King's Fund Centre grant funded: that we had funded many extra staff, as well as totally revamping whole wards. This was untrue. We felt strongly that it was up to the health authorities, who at the start of the project were service providers, to fund establishment posts, including new posts concerned with service delivery. Our grant-giving was designed to support internal development posts and even with these, some commitment from the health authority was expected.

All the posts were different, reflecting the individual needs of each NDU, but the new roles had common development responsibilities.

The people in the new posts were expected to act as change agents. Their task was to help the team bring about a cycle of change or to foster change agency in others by bringing new skills or knowledge to the team or to reinforce existing skills. For example, there were two research posts (Joy Warren at Weymouth and Barbara Sheppard at Brighton) where, in addition to bringing their expertise to bear on specific issues, they helped individual nurses undertake their own research and evaluation projects.

The posts were also expected to be developmental for the people in them, helping them develop themselves as well as nursing; perhaps this is best illustrated by the two new development staff nurse posts at Southport (Karen Wright and Jenny McGuire). Each post had designated time for an experienced staff nurse to undertake project work related to the NDU. In some cases the work involved helping the rest of the team to introduce a new practice, such as Karen's work on documenting care. Sometimes the work was more an individual research project, such as Jenny's work on nutrition. All the posts were developmental to the wider field of nursing in that they created and tested more options for clinical posts, even where they sounded very similar to existing posts or created new working relationships. An example of this was to be found in Brighton in the relationship between Barbara, who was not a nurse but an experienced researcher, and the NDU team.

The posts also made a statement to the host hospital and health authority about the value of development and the importance of planned change, situated against a backdrop which could have been hostile to these values – where costs, closures and frozen posts appeared to be the dominant concern.

Introducing these new roles was not without difficulties. There were misunderstandings about their purpose, which led to difficulties in maintaining boundaries. For example, one of the development staff nurses, who was graded as an F for her clinical development responsibilities, was asked to provide managerial cover for the hospital in evenings and weekends like other F grade nurses. A lecturer practitioner who was a joint appointee between the hospital and university found her clinical role eroded by the demands of the educational component. At the outset of the project, one NDU leader faced increasing demands from the central organisation and chief nurse's office. It seemed hard for those outside the NDU to appreciate the focused nature of the work; and because there were few development posts in the wider organisation, there was a tendency to try to spread the expertise widely, jeopardising the focus on the NDU.

Nurses, both in the new posts and in other leadership roles in the NDUs, faced increased demands from internal and external work, frequently involving them in work outside their regular hours. At the King's Fund Centre we wanted to create realistic roles so that developing nursing could be undertaken by any nurse. We did not want to create 'supernurses' to perform Herculean feats.

A third difficulty was clarifying the new roles, including my own, related to the NDU team. New posts, with no predetermined place in the nursing team, challenged the existing order. Jane Salvage and I had tried to pre-empt this by questioning lines of responsibility and accountability that appeared vague or ambiguous; but even when they were clear, there were difficulties. Aspects of leadership had to be renegotiated, and the work which related to the NDU as distinct from the ward had to be divided. A balance had to be struck between people wanting to undertake aspects of leadership because they felt it belonged to them, and new types of leadership from people whom the nursing team felt could best support them in this work. Ironing out these issues was fraught for everyone in the new posts. It was emotionally draining and tiring for the whole team and appeared to be stultifying, blocking some developments early on in the project.

These difficulties were minimised in the early stages by clear job descriptions and specification of personal qualities required in filling the post, and lines of responsibility. These had to be thought through carefully, reflecting the local situation. In Southport, for example, when we were developing the leader role, one of the managers was very keen on a prototype developed elsewhere. In some ways this distracted us from developing a role appropriate to the NDU, although it was later resolved. In the same NDU the F grade development staff nurse posts were relatively easy to describe as no prototype existed. Throughout the project constant negotiation of the boundaries of the work helped to sort out misunderstandings external to the NDU and to allow the new roles to develop their full potential. This is illustrated in Brighton where Brenda Hawkey, the NDU leader, initially had no designated time for development work. With support from the rest of her team she was able to balance the demands of providing care with the role of NDU leader. As the development work increased it was possible to negotiate designated time for Brenda's development work. She retained clinical involvement, but some of her time was dedicated to development support to those giving care.

In getting the new roles right, it was essential to pay attention to the emotional content of the work: the threats we pose to others in our new roles and that others pose to us. This was also vital for helping NDU nurses deal with people in new roles throughout the organisation. This work is never easy; by its very nature it makes us slightly uncomfortable with ourselves. It is difficult to acknowledge that a colleague threatens us because she seems to have more skills, knowledge or popularity, or that I threaten her in a similar way. Such threats arose not only from the introduction of new posts, but also from the staff's changing roles as they strove to develop a new form of nursing.

Empowering relationships

Empowerment and autonomy for nurses and patients are central to the philosophy of the 'New Nursing', but what do they mean in practice? This patient from Brighton NDU, talking to Barbara Sheppard as part of her action research with the NDU team, illustrates the relationship between empowered nurses and empowered patients (Sheppard 1991). Empowering patients means transferring to them the sources of power – knowledge, skills and resources, and eventually letting go.

> Well, X in particular gave you confidence. A big strong girl – you could have a joke with her, but she could be quite strict if she thought you were doing something wrong. She could give you a damn good telling off! I admitted one day to her that when I went to the toilet by myself that I hung on the wash basin to position myself and I said, 'Don't be surprised if the whole wash basin collapses on the floor some time.' She said, 'You haven't told me, have you?' And I said, 'No I haven't.' She used to pull my leg about it. 'How's the wash basin, David? Still on the wall is it?' And I'd say, 'Yes, very handy isn't it,' and she'd say, 'Well I've never heard of it, have I!'
>
> That sort of touch like that suits a patient like me very well. And I took good care that I didn't pull it off the wall but I said to her, 'Look, I've found this particular loo most convenient for manoeuvring about but I do cling to the wash basin.' She just laughed. She was a good judge of a patient. Some would have forbidden it. Others, like me, she knew. 'It's all right, he's OK. He won't kill himself or fetch the wash basin off the wall and if he does, I'll have to put it back on again.' But trusting like that.

As I worked with the units I saw different types of personal and professional development which helped to empower patients and nurses. Nurses developed new skills to improve the range and depth of clinical interventions they could offer and to equip themselves to lead developments in their units and in the wider organisation. They reorganised the delivery of care so that decision-making was devolved to the patient and to those closest to him/her and his relatives and they evolved new relations with their nursing colleagues and the multidisciplinary team.

New skills and knowledge

In the NDUs nurses explored their need for new skills and new areas of knowledge as they tried to develop their practice. The variety of new areas was vast, ranging from developing new techniques for moving patients to the more expressive skills of health education and counselling. A distinctive development for nurses in general hospitals was working with patients in groups; two NDUs had such goals in their earliest objectives. In Brighton, Sheena McKenzie, carrying out a research project on group reminiscence therapy as a rehabilitation tool, highlighted the importance of understanding, planning and facilitating group processes (McKenzie 1991).

The type of skills developed in the units varied, but it was possible to identify with the NDU leaders some common areas for development. Joint workshops were held over the three years, focusing on evaluation, time management, personal power and assertion, presentation skills, and learning the lessons of the closure of the Oxford NDU. Some were more successful than others. Despite two seminars on evaluation with expert contributions, much more was learned experientially in the units through undertaking small evaluative projects.

Reorganising care delivery

Reorganisation of the delivery of care also aimed to empower patients and staff. As with the new formal roles, reorganising care delivery – whether to primary nursing or to a variant of team nursing – had considerable impact on existing roles, not always as predicted. This is well illustrated in the senior nurse's account in Case Study 6.1.

Case Study 6.1
The senior nurse's story

I first became a ward sister 11 years ago and have been a ward-based senior nurse for the past five years. When we started primary nursing little thought was given to my changing role. We concentrated on the changing roles of the other trained staff.

We decided at the beginning that all change would be decided democratically, so while I did not always agree with everything, I did not deliberately attempt to hinder the developments. Although I was happy for us to progress, the ward previously ran very smoothly and at times I found it difficult to understand why there was a need for change.

At the beginning I worked as a coordinator to try to ensure the smooth running of the ward. Change was gradual and in the early stages the difficulties caused by our lack of preparation for my role change were not unearthed. However, within months the need for a ward coordinator seemed unnecessary and it was then that we realised we had not thought through my role long term. This was a very daunting experience. Not only was there the feeling of not being needed, but I found guiding and supporting the staff through change very stressful and I longed for the good old days!

After much thought and discussion in the team I took on the role of an associate nurse. The role of primary nurse, although appealing, would not be possible as too much time would be spent away from the patients by my other duties as senior nurse. Being an associate nurse proved more difficult than anticipated. Subconsciously, I found myself taking over and acting as the primary nurse. Retrospectively, I can see that during that period I probably hindered the development of the primary nurse by not allowing her the time or space to develop.

With an unexpected ward closure, we had three weeks before reopening our new ward to look critically at where we were, where we would like to go and in particular what my role should be. This time for reflection was invaluable. I realised that when working in a group as an associate nurse, I should support and facilitate for the group to progress as a whole, and I should not be so interested in the glory of who instigated the care. Old habits die hard. Perhaps my new role can be best clarified using four headings:

1. *Patient care*: I am involved in the delivery of patient care. Decisions on

the prescribing of care are often collective as a group, although the primary nurse has the final say on how the care is to be delivered.

2. *Management*: Because I am no longer the central person prescribing care, doing the ward rounds and being the person everyone wants to talk to, I am able to allow myself planned time to prepare for meetings and fulfil my hospital commitments. At first I felt guilty using work time for writing references, doing the off-duty, etc. – many of the things that as a traditional sister I ended up doing at home because I did not want staff to say, 'Sister's in the office.' Now it is accepted that I need this time and the staff have a greater appreciation of what a senior nurse does.

3. *Teaching*: Before the introduction of primary nursing it proved almost impossible to commit myself to a teaching programme. Now I have more time available to work with and teach individuals. I am also able to allow myself time to learn and develop new skills. Initially, it was threatening to admit that others might know more than I did, but gradually I have come to shed this stereotype image that the sister is an all-knowing, all-doing, all-being person.

At first there was a little competition between the primary nurses. They still wanted to prove themselves to the sister and saw asking for advice as a failure. Now, secure in their new roles, they frequently ask how I would solve a problem.

4. *Personal development*: Like the other qualified staff, I too have completed a learning contract – something else that was threatening and difficult to accept. I have been able to direct my development in areas previously alien to me.

Giving up the reins sounds much easier than it actually is. If I'm honest, not being the centre of attention and having my finger permanently on what I thought was the pulse proved to be difficult and made me feel vulnerable and defenceless. The support and understanding of the staff and my manager has made life more tolerable, and working directly and closely with a group of patients has certainly compensated for the heartache along the way.

Another NDU in our network had carefully approached the introduction of primary nursing – they felt it would really challenge their abilities and could create tension in the team. In the event, they made a relatively smooth transition to primary nursing. They then attempted to introduce the self-administration of medication to the ward, which they felt well equipped to do. This was much more difficult; despite a fundamental belief that patients could and should control their own treatments, the nurses found the change more threatening.

Each one of us needs to be aware of our own prejudices and feelings; to whom do we feel most uncomfortable about introducing self-medication and why? We also need to be able to allow experiment and risk-taking by the patient. Taking responsibility means taking responsibility for the possibility of failure, but not for failure itself. Moreover, becoming empowered is not a final state. Most of us experienced times when we felt we could conquer Everest and others when even getting to the foothills felt impossible. Recognising when we might feel undermined was half the battle.

New relations with colleagues

Changes in working practices also have an impact on team relations and patterns of leadership, within and outside the NDU. Recently, a health visitor commented that the NDU was dependent on nurses working as a team and this posed particular difficulties for health visitors, who had to think themselves back into the 'family of nursing'. Philosophically, the team nature of the NDU arises from two sources: the humanistic principle that humans are naturally social beings; and the strong tradition of creative teamwork in nursing itself. That the NDU is a team concept is not incompatible with the development of individual nurses, but central to it. As the health visitor observed, the team concept is important in the NDU but extends across the family of nursing.

Teamwork has been vital in promoting and securing changes in practice. In some of the units, active team-building has taken place. Brenda Hawkey from Brighton NDU noted that each time a new member joined the team a new cycle of team-building occurred and dedicated time was required for this. Although the NDUs have retained staff, other local factors have influenced team membership. In one hospital the number of elderly care wards was reduced; staff from the four closed wards were redeployed on the remaining two wards, one being the NDU. They were often distressed by the closure of their wards, loss of 'their' patients and grief for the loss of their roles; their feelings of powerlessness were to some extent heightened by the NDU culture, where change was a constant and the existing staff did not have conventional roles. Considerable effort was required to build the team.

Some units have used the team as a forum for resolving difficulties. In Brighton NDU, the clinical psychologist has worked regularly with the team, while nurses in West Dorset NDU set up support groups.

Working in an NDU can be particularly stressful for student nurses, who are transitory members of the team. At the beginning of the project, students complained that their development was no longer the sole focus of teaching and learning on the ward; as the patterns of work changed, some experienced a loss of status as they increasingly shared with qualified staff the role of giving direct patient care; some found the shift towards patients' individual needs and away from ward routines disorienting and anxiety-provoking – what was expected of them? However, others felt positive about the NDU.

Clinical practice is a complex activity, requiring clinical leadership at the bedside in order to analyse situations, determine priorities, offer choices to patients, support them in decision-making and choose ways of delivering care most effectively. These skills are transferable. If nurses have the skill to do this at the bedside, they also have the potential to do it at team level and beyond. Nursing brings to the organisation 'endemic leadership'. However, traditional ways of working are deeply embedded. General management means the locus of power has changed, but not necessarily the flow of management, which remains top-down. While generating new patterns of leadership, nurses are operating in a traditional and sometimes stifling climate. This sometimes leads to a tension between the different types of leadership required for the NDU. The project usually started life with someone advocating for the NDU in the organisation, someone with a high profile in the NDU and outside it. As leadership skills in the NDU are mobilised, different patterns of leadership evolve and contribute to the richness of the work.

Supportive networks

At the start of the project we foresaw a unique opportunity to foster peer support among the four NDUs, particularly the leaders and the network members. We organised a series of workshops for the four NDUs and some events for those in the wider network to provide input on topics common to the NDUs and to provide space for people to share their experiences. Everyone in the units seemed as enthusiastic as us to work in this way.

It soon became apparent, however, that nurses found it extremely hard to discuss their difficulties, whether they were from the four NDUS or the wider network. For example, I invited two nurses from the north of England and two nurses from a London ward to discuss their plans. In our telephone discussions both groups highlighted their problems in getting recognition and management support. When arranging the visit I asked if they would mind my inviting some other nurses who were also trying to get an NDU off the ground so that we could compare notes; they agreed. However, at the meeting they revealed few of these issues, concentrating on describing to each other their achievements, despite my efforts to steer the discussion towards thornier problems. When the nurses from the north left to catch their train, the London nurses started to tell me about the threat of closure they felt their unit was under. When I asked why they hadn't raised the issue in the wider group, they said they did not want to dampen the others' enthusiasm for the project.

Although the NDU projects came from different settings and distinct cultures, they shared the experience of changes in the wider health service. As a result, all four at some point perceived themselves as under threat of closure or a severely curtailed existence as an NDU. Individually, the leaders looked to me for reassurance that they were not the only NDU experiencing this or other problems, but once they met in a group they would deny that there were shared experiences, either directly or by failing to participate. While the NDU leaders had considerable leadership and facilitation skills in their own units, they seemed unwilling to take responsibility for this in the wider group of the four NDUs. More recently the leaders have started meeting independently to support each other, so perhaps the lesson is that these things cannot be rushed; group processes are complex.

Internal plans for individual development

The development and education opportunities for NDU staff increased with the award of the King's Fund Centre grant. However, in the first years, the number of formal study days remained relatively low, with staff enjoying a range of 1.5 – 2.9 study days per person per year in three of the units, while staff in the fourth unit had 5.7 – 6 study days each (Turner-Shaw and Bosanquet 1993). The number of days is important, especially in terms of cost, but does not reflect the variety and ingenuity of the units in creating individual and collective learning opportunities. Many of these later became an integral part of ward activities.

Each NDU has its own strategy for developing individual nurses. In Camberwell NDU painstaking work was done on personal development plans for staff (Herbert and Evans 1991), while West Dorset invited trainers from the Samaritans to help them develop their interpersonal skills. Different units explored a variety of approaches to staff development which reflected the organisational culture, history and priorities of the unit. As with changes in practice, new ways of learning and development became the norm and were often seen as unremarkable by those in the projects. Creativity and hard work in the NDUs were boosted by the practical advantage of having a small grant dedicated to staff development, but in all the NDUs staff generated other funds for their development needs.

Nurses in the NDUs have had an opportunity to deepen their understanding of how they nurse by looking at practice intensively and challenging it. This has not always been comfortable. Admitting that something we have done for years could be done better if we had new or better skills can be very threatening. It can also be very cathartic, exploring how we can manage rather than control.

Small, manageable evaluative projects have helped the NDUs to identify how they nurse and how they need to develop, individually and as a team. Some of these projects have been written up in journals and in other publications (e.g. Black 1992). They provided individual development for the person leading the project and led to practice-based learning for the team. When one primary nurse wished to demonstrate different pain-relieving techniques, the ward became a living laboratory with nurses as guinea pigs using buckets of ice to induce pain and to evaluate how effectively the therapies worked.

Staff set themselves high standards and could be too hard on themselves. Mandy Norton, a staff nurse in West Dorset NDU, questioned to what extent the assessment of a patient at risk of developing pressure sores informed nursing practice. The Norton scale (no relation) was used to assess patients on admission. Mandy decided to look at her own patients; all were assessed using the Norton scale and those at risk had a component of their care plan recognising the problem. However, the care prescribed was not personalised and the use of pressure-relieving aids was haphazard. Mandy was self-critical, pointing out that her tiny sample and the use of her own patients reduced the objectivity of the study. However, it was just these factors which contributed to the success of the project in bringing about change. She increased the team's awareness about this area of practice, informed her colleagues about good practice and minimised resistance to change by exposing her own practice to critique. In the process she developed her own skills in literature review, auditing care plans, observation, recording data, writing up her results and presenting them. This work will be repeated, with some adaptation, as part of the NDU audit.

Nurses in each NDU have undertaken similar small projects related to a variety of clinical issues such as wound care, pain relief, nutrition, the use of a nursing model and group reminiscence. In undertaking such work they have developed a variety of new skills. Some are research-related, such as questionnaire design and interviewing techniques. Others concern how to bring about change, such as time management. One of the successes has been that any nurse in the NDU, part-time or full-time, enrolled or registered, has been able to undertake such project work. Sometimes it was difficult getting the balance right between individual projects and the common enterprise. In one unit where many small projects were started at the outset, some floundered as the work grew out of proportion; it was difficult to get support for a project when every nurse was distracted by her own. Integrating the project into the overall work is necessary and may change the goals of other projects.

The success of the projects depended on the support available from the new development posts; the parameters and focus of the research – 'small is beautiful', generally speaking; and designated time made available by colleagues' flexibility and money from the Department of Health, which paid to release a staff nurse for 7.5 hours a week to work on evaluation.

A successful strategy?

When I started writing this account I had in the back of my mind this question: How do I measure success or failure? The NDUs themselves will be tested in a variety of ways. Internally, the nurses will evaluate whether patient care improves; Janet Turner-Shaw's evaluation for the Department of Health (Turner-Shaw and Bosanquet 1993) tells us to what extent the units are NDUs; and the success of the overall project may be judged by the impact it makes on policy decisions about developing nursing. However, it is more difficult to assess to what extent the strategy for developing nurses has been a success. I cannot claim credit for the skill, enthusiasm and industry of nurses in the units as development workers in their own projects.

There have been moments of despair, when preparation and effort failed to generate enthusiasm for some joint venture from my colleagues in the NDUs. But there have also been great moments – proof for me that the strategy works. Sometimes it is watching a staff nurse skilfully facilitate her own team in moving forward on a particular development issue. At other times it is observing a nurse make a successful presentation to the chief executive and health authority member about how the team will address the next stage of a project. Sometimes the successful partnership is even more fleeting, such as the day an NDU leader telephoned me before going into a meeting with her manager to run through with me how she would play it. These successes may seem small but they are the stuff of empowerment.

References

Black G (ed.) (1992), *Nursing Development Units: Work in Progress*. London: King's Fund Centre.

Herbert R and Evans A (1991) Staff appraisal and development. *Senior Nurse* **11**(6): 9–11.

McKenzie S (1991) A positive force. *Nursing the Elderly* **3**(3): 22–24.

Sheppard B (1991) *Patients and Carers: Perceptions of Being on Homeward*. Unpublished interim research report.

Turner-Shaw J and Bosanquet N (1993) *Nursing Development Units: A Way to Develop Nurses and Nursing*. London: King's Fund Centre.

CHAPTER 7

Doing Development Work

Gillian Black

This chapter looks at development work and some of the issues that arose during the course of the King's Fund Centre's NDU programme. It is not an attempt to provide a comprehensive guide to change in nursing, but to give some insights into what we learned as the project progressed. I have included examples of techniques which I found helpful, so it is also a 'tool box', although not a definitive one.

None of us involved with the project came to the collaborative venture of development work empty-handed. All had a record of introducing change and good and bad experiences to share. As the project progressed we all had the opportunity of trying out new ways of managing the cycle of change, developing new skills to do this and sometimes jettisoning long-cherished beliefs.

Learning from other people was important for me. For example, once the units had been selected, Liz Winn, a project worker (not a nurse) in the King's Fund Centre's primary health care programme, helped me identify the key components of the contract for development work agreed with each unit. Facilitative and reflective supervision came from my manager and from an external supervisor, who actively listened to descriptions of my work, challenged my assumptions and helped me to evolve new ways of looking at problems. This support was enhanced by in-house and external courses for King's Fund Centre staff; of particular note were courses on consultancy skills and presentation skills.

Development work and consultancy

In Chapter 1, change was compared to a journey where the travelling is as important as the destination. Development work is the input of skills, knowledge and support to help make that journey. It is an integral part of most leadership roles and is part of all management. However, it takes different forms (and may be called different things) depending on the philosophy which underpins the approach and the relationship of the development worker with the people undertaking the change. In many circumstances the terms consultancy and development work are interchangeable.

Consultancy/development work can be regarded as occurring along at least two different axes: from inside the system to outside the system (see Figure 7.1), from empowering people to do their own development work to doing it for them.

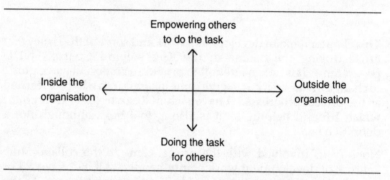

Figure 7.1 Development work and consultancy

Our development work with the projects was characterised by several features, as follows:

- King's Fund Centre project workers are involved over a longer period than in many other types of consultancy despite being 'outside' the organisation. This provides opportunities for developing better, long-term support systems for managing change. Because the process of change was of as much interest to us as the end-result, we were keen to share with colleagues in the NDUs the processes that enable the 'journey' to progress; making explicit what we thought was happening.

- The King's Fund Centre has a record of working in this way with health service projects and therefore provides opportunities for cross-fertilisation. This occurred several times during the first years of the project. For example, Southport NDU was interested in active involvement of carers in their plans for development and we were able to provide specific expertise via the King's Fund Centre's Carers Project.

- We believed that nurses, once empowered to do so, could find their own solutions to health service problems. We were therefore anxious not to prescribe solutions but to work with the NDUs to build a vision of what nursing care could achieve and identify how to realise it.

- We recognised that 'support' came in different guises. Sometimes the best support is to relieve someone of something burdensome or to bring in additional expertise. While we were involved in a longer-term piece of development work, we also enlisted consultants who, working with us on a shorter time-scale, adopted a similarly empowering approach. The willingness of other experienced nurses – practitioners, managers, researchers and academics as well as management consultants – to give their time and energies (often for minimal payment) to the project as a whole or to specific NDUs was an exciting aspect of the work.

At the beginning of the project I met staff in the four NDUs to discuss how we would work together, what my role should be and how I would relate to the team. There was considerable anxiety in the projects about the implications of the King's Fund Centre grant and it was not clear to staff how I might be able to help them. From our discussions I drew up a draft contract which suggested what my role should be and asked them to review it. We identified that I might work with staff in a number of different ways:

- Guiding the project through developing and agreeing objectives, planning a programme of work and reviewing progress
- Acting as a sounding board and helping to consider developments as they emerged
- Acting as a consultant on professional, policy and management issues and on the change process
- Discussing how to create a climate conducive to nursing developments
- Supporting NDU staff in dissemination of developments to other disciplines, the health authority and the profession
- Contributing experience of other nursing development work, lessons from other NDUs and knowledge from the literature
- Providing shared learning experiences between the four NDUs
- Generating contacts with other health authorities undertaking similar activities

I undertook some of these activities in each unit but there was a different emphasis in each, and my contribution changed over the period of three years. There were occasional bursts of activity in a particular unit, usually in response to a request from the NDU leader for me to take on a specific role.

Facilitation for patients and nurses

Theoretically, it might be possible to divide the types of skill and knowledge that nurses need to bring about change into those required for the development of practice itself, e.g. clinical skills; the abilities required for bringing about organisational change in the NDU and in the wider organisation; and the ability to deal with new roles, relationships and teamwork. In my experience the divisions are artificial. This was brought home to me early on in the project, when I sat in on the weekly meeting of the ward multidisciplinary team in one of the NDUs. My observations of one nurse's role in that meeting are given in Case Study 7.1.

Case Study 7.1
The facilitated multidisciplinary ward meeting

I observed a nurse putting the case for a patient's right to try to return home as he wished, against the view held by all the other disciplines that he should be transferred to a rest home.

The nurse in question facilitated the group throughout the meeting, paying attention to the group dynamics and the organisational politics that underpinned them. In fact, she participated only a little in the information – giving activity that surrounded discussion of the other patients, using questions and seeking opinions of other members of the team to form a rounded picture of each patient. Her body language showed her to be relaxed and confident and while saying little, she appeared interested in what others were saying, only taking notes when they had finished speaking. When it came to discussing the patient who wished to go home, she drew on her clinical knowledge and her knowledge of him to make his case, but without denying the risk that both the patient and the team would be taking. She spoke quietly and unemotionally. When the team began to discuss the issues she reflected back to them what they were saying, gently challenging their assumptions. The team agreed to give active support to the patient's discharge home and the whole tenor of the discussion changed to a collaborative planning exercise on what help might be offered to this patient. The outcome of this part of the meeting could have been so different if the nurse had not paid attention throughout to the processes of the meeting, or if she had displayed impatience or anger with her colleagues, who from her point of view were ignoring a patient's rights, or if she had not had the clinical knowledge or the knowledge of the patient's situation to support her case.

An appreciation of how people feel in a variety of situations and an understanding of roles and relationships, plus skills and tools to use this knowledge carefully and ethically, are vital to bringing about changes in practice which may on the surface appear simple. Managing or helping other people to move forward, whether in an informal, one-to-one situation or in a formal, larger meeting, demands more than the technical knowledge and skill which may have brought you into the meeting in the first place. It is not necessary to be the person in charge to facilitate a meeting. Anyone can take responsibility for this and help the meeting along. In a group where all the members are facilitating each other it is likely that considerable progress will be made.

There are at least three streams of activity that need to be managed if the group (which could just be you and one other person) is to move from its present position to a new position, as illustrated in Figure 7.2.

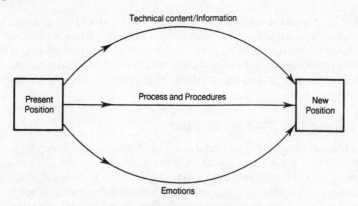

Figure 7.2 Facilitating a move forward

1. *The technical content* consists of the raw information being brought to bear on the issue being discussed. Sometimes progress can be blocked by inadequate, irrelevant or complex information. In the example given, the information about the patient's abilities,

home situation, what the patient wanted and the risks helped the meeting move on.

2. *The process stream of activity* is concerned with how the meeting is managed. It includes checking how much time everyone has for this discussion and agreeing what sort of record is to be made and to whom it will be available. Does everyone in the meeting have the opportunity to make their point? Is everyone aware of the agenda? Are key points summarised and verified before moving on? The process can be blocked right from the start by uncomfortable seating arrangements. Being facilitative means taking responsibility for overcoming those blocks, for trying to make it comfortable for everyone to participate. In the example given, the nurse reflected back to the other disciplines what they were saying to raise their awareness of the assumptions they were making. Challenging them directly might have blocked the process.

3. *The emotional stream of activity* is primarily concerned with the management of feelings that the meeting is generating among the participants. Body language and voice changes may indicate how people are feeling. In the case described, the nurse demonstrated how she valued other people's opinions and gained reciprocity by doing this; when she had something to say, her opinion was valued.

Thinking about meetings in this way can be useful in planning a meeting and for debriefing following a meeting. It helps to focus on what information will be required, from me or from others; what sort of processes might keep the discussion moving and what might block it; and what emotions might be generated in me or in others.

Making the changes happen

At the outset each NDU had drawn up a plan of work as part of its application for a King's Fund Centre grant. Once the project was under way the units set about making their overall vision a reality. This involved setting goals and priorities and determining shorter-term action plans. In the first year I often found myself questioning plans that looked too ambitious. Written, short-term action plans were helpful when a team hit a low point. There was a natural ebb and flow to the development work, with staff making considerable changes in practice and then consolidating them. However, there were times when the impetus was lost, sometimes because of events outside the unit; threats to the unit, such as ward closures; or overload of demand, especially on the NDU leader. It was then possible via the plans to look back on what had been achieved. Staff in the units were often surprised by the ground they had covered – innovations became the usual way of doing things and therefore were invisible to those in the units.

One of the unforeseen factors affecting the project was the high turnover of managers supporting the four NDUs. Of the initial six people who made up the group of NDU managers, only two now remain in a post related to their NDU, while three out of the four NDUs have gained a new executive nurse – none of whom was involved in the project at the outset. These changes required a constant revisiting of the vision of the NDU to enlist new managers' support for the concept and to incorporate their aspirations into the overall picture.

In some ways this group has experienced more changes in roles and relationships than those in the NDUs. Understanding this was important to the development work. The nurse managers have often been very isolated, their strengths are not valued by the wider management team and they have to juggle with unrealistic expectations from the nurses they manage.

The changes in the four NDUs and their host organisations highlighted the need for nurses to manage in a variety of different directions, including managing their bosses. Case Study 7.2 illustrates how one NDU leader and I worked together to address how the organisational changes affected her relations with managers. The case study shows that successful managers are those who manage relationships up the system as well as down it. This means recognising that different managers have different work styles and aptitudes and that effective boss–subordinate relationships depend on the recognition of mutual dependence between fallible human beings. Managing the mutual dependence requires a good understanding of your boss and yourself, especially regarding strengths, weakness, work styles and needs. It also requires you to use this information to develop and manage a healthy working relationship, compatible with both people's work styles and assets, characterised by mutual expectations and meeting the most critical needs of the other person (Gabarro and Kotter 1980).

Case Study 7.2

Support for a clinical leader: a view from one NDU

The second year of the King's Fund grant was a particularly busy and stressful year for me as clinical leader. The change in my role, while welcome, had increased my workload enormously. I was now trying to fulfil my clinical role, fully rostered; I had taken on greater managerial responsibility following our manager's departure; and within the unit greater changes were required as the team took forward projects.

The NDU at this time was arousing interest and gaining respect from within and outside the health authority; more visits and enquiries were being supported. The success of the unit was creating a huge amount of work and I began to feel unable to fulfil all aspects of my role.

All the team were very supportive and suggested one day a week off the rota, for 'business' and development work. Despite a concerted effort, the demands of the ward often prevented my achieving supernumerary status although the days I was off the rota were beneficial. Offers of administrative support were made by my new manager and the chief nursing adviser, but they never really materialised.

By summer 1991 the annual report was completed. It included several observations on the amount of extra work now required of me and the need for administrative assistance.

Meanwhile threats of closure of wards loomed and our unit remained a likely target. Staff were generally feeling insecure for the first time in years, despite their continued enthusiasm for development. Gill Black suggested that the two managers directly involved with the NDU should meet with us to agree some ways of providing further support for me.

I remember feeling relieved at this point, but also apprehensive. I was aware that the directorate nurse manager did not fully appreciate the amount and importance of the work which was being generated by the NDU, or the difference between my duties and those of an 'ordinary' ward sister.

At my next meeting with Gill, I indicated my despair at trying unsuccessfully to fulfil all my goals and convince my manager of the importance of the work. I remember being very grateful that Gill had come with a very positive attitude. While I found it hard to lift my own emotions, it had the effect of spurring me into some kind of action – if only acknowledging that the workload was overburdening me and not that I was inadequate.

We discussed my role in terms of the three areas: development, management and direct care to patients. We agreed to concentrate our presentation to the two managers on 'development'. Gill suggested we illustrate the considerable change in my role on a flip chart.

She also felt it might be useful to acknowledge how these two managers might be feeling and ways we could enhance the meeting by showing an understanding of their difficulties. We felt that one remained committed to the NDU but was overburdened by a new job and that the other, also in a new post, was perhaps looking for management approval but none the less wanted to be part of what was a successful quality initiative.

The first joint meeting with the managers was a little tense despite being held in the familiar ward setting. I felt very nervous about it and was glad to have Gill's support. I was concerned that both managers would feel threatened. I remember feeling cold and anxious at the meeting and let Gill do most of the talking – then afterwards felt guilty about it. I was a little worried by some of the responses to the presentation. It was suggested that the work I was doing should be carried out by all G grade sisters. Gill was assertive and gave good examples of work undertaken by me which would not be considered by other sisters, such as carrying through the implementation from the action research.

It was certainly not a warm meeting; I felt some reserve between the two managers. One was obviously trying to be fair, admitting support from the organisation had been less than promised and acknowledging an obligation to support the unit in some other way. The other manager offered to take it back to directorate level. Neither offered any tangible support at this encounter.

Gill and I met after the meeting to discuss our tactics. We both agreed it had been useful to plan carefully. I felt I would need Gill's support at the next stage as my confidence had waned. I realised then my lack of negotiating skills at management level. Gill remained positive about a successful outcome to the proposal we agreed to put forward.

My next meeting with Gill was very productive. I had given a great deal of thought to the problem and discussed it further with one of the managers concerned. He pledged support in the form of administrative help. Gill and I planned that we would ask the other manager for supernumerary time and replacement staff for me to take three days off the rota. These would include time spent working with nurses on the unit plus appraisal time, and would also allow me to concentrate for uninterrupted periods on NDU work – coordination of projects, facilitating staff, arranging visits, giving seminars, and so on.

The meeting planned between the four of us took place without one of the managers but achieved our objective and left all three of us feeling satisfied. Some areas were still unsolved such as office space and these are being worked on now.

The outcome was a highly successful proposal, with compromises being made on both sides but, throughout, respect for each other's position. Gill's interventions were skilful and timely, but most importantly she took some of the pressure off me when I was feeling vulnerable and enabled me to move forward in my objectives.

Having a shared vision is not enough. Knowing how to get there is also necessary; one useful method is force field analysis. NDU network members attended a workshop on introducing change in clinical settings in September 1990 to learn how to use this method from Stevie Holland of GO Education. The tool is especially useful when you know where you want to go but are stuck or making unacceptably slow progress. It is based on the work of Kurt Lewin (1951), who noticed that in organisations there were always forces operating that would, in an ideal world, bring about change. These he called 'driving forces'. He also observed that there were forces likely to inhibit change: 'restraining forces'. These two sets of forces working against each other tend to create a 'dynamic equilibrium' which shifts if either the driving forces or restraining forces are altered (see Figure 7.3).

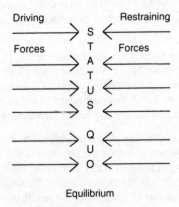

Figure 7.3 Force field concept

Lewin observed that for a situation to change it was not enough to encourage the driving forces; the restraining forces needed to be addressed and reduced or removed. Those trying to bring about change commonly direct their energies to pushing harder for change. This may well increase resistance from others and exhaust and demoralise the change agents. Reducing the restraining forces may be a more creative way, both personally and organisationally, to unfreeze the situation.

We used force field analysis as a group method in the workshop but it can be used as an individual and personal method of assessing the need for change. If you are using it as a group method you will need to consider how it is facilitated. It is quite time-consuming to do as a group but this should be weighed against its efficacy in determining a realistic action plan to which people will be committed. Once they are familiar with the method, it becomes easier to use.

There are five stages involved in force field analysis. The first is to map out the 'field'. The group or individual needs to identify the problem, the desired outcome and the present situation (the current equilibrium). The second stage is to identify the main driving forces for the proposed change and the main forces restraining it. The forces may be social, psychological or physical; real or imagined. Factors which we may consider imaginary may appear real to dissatisfied parties. Rather than aiming to get it perfect, brainstorm all the things that keep the situation as it is, that maintain the current equilibrium. You can then organise them into forces for change, the driving forces and the forces against change, the restraining forces. There may be a similar content of opposing forces and it is helpful to arrange these opposite each other. Where this is not the case, it does not matter in what order they are placed as long as they are on the appropriate force side. I have taken an example from the workshop, where a group of nurses looked at the handover of patient care between nurses. They described the field and forces as illustrated in Figure 7.3.

The next stage is to gauge the strength of the different forces. In a personal example this is relatively simple, as the forces often arouse deep feelings. In a group it is possible to gauge how strong the different forces are by asking each member to rate how strong the forces are for them. Each person should consider each force and ascribe to it a value:

0 = not relevant/no force
1 = low force
2 = medium force
3 = high force

By adding up the scores it is possible to consider the strength of the forces. In Figure 7.4 below, honesty was the strongest force pushing for change, while fear of breaching confidentiality was the strongest force restraining change. The scores are the small numbers in brackets by each force.

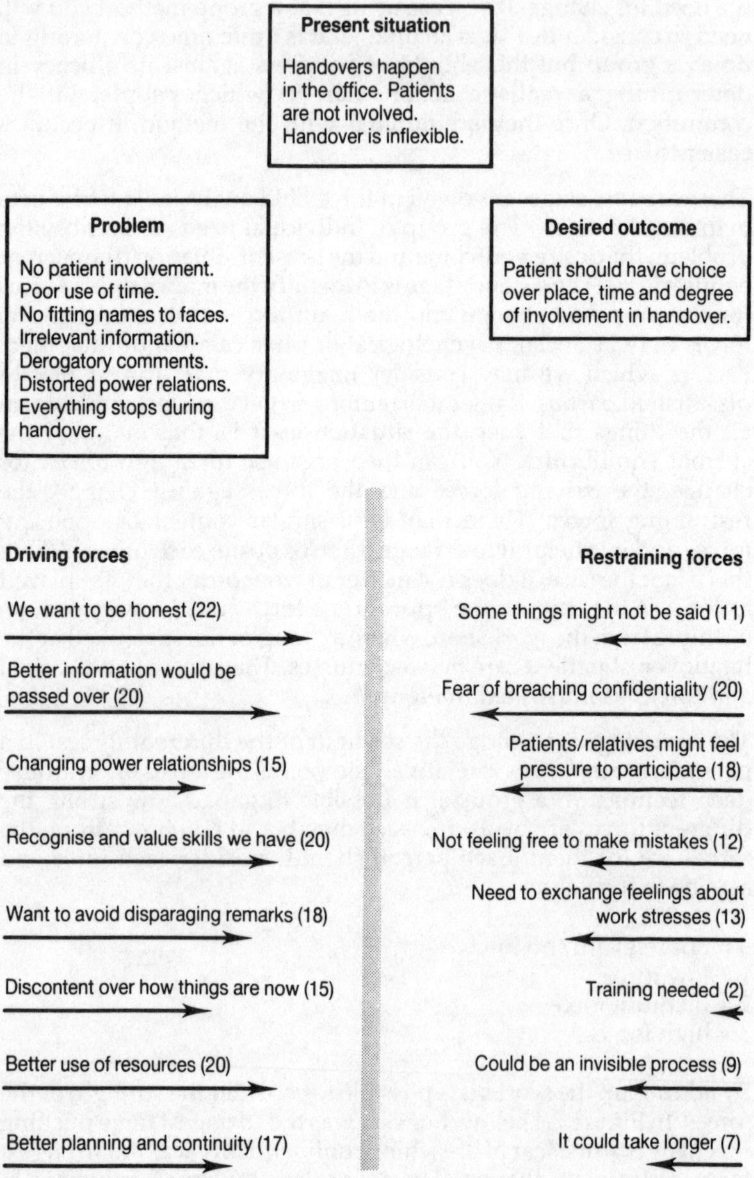

Present situation

Handovers happen
in the office. Patients
are not involved.
Handover is inflexible.

Problem

No patient involvement.
Poor use of time.
No fitting names to faces.
Irrelevant information.
Derogatory comments.
Distorted power relations.
Everything stops during
handover.

Desired outcome

Patient should have choice
over place, time and degree
of involvement in handover.

Driving forces

We want to be honest (22)

Better information would be
passed over (20)

Changing power relationships (15)

Recognise and value skills we have (20)

Want to avoid disparaging remarks (18)

Discontent over how things are now (15)

Better use of resources (20)

Better planning and continuity (17)

Restraining forces

Some things might not be said (11)

Fear of breaching confidentiality (20)

Patients/relatives might feel
pressure to participate (18)

Not feeling free to make mistakes (12)

Need to exchange feelings about
work stresses (13)

Training needed (2)

Could be an invisible process (9)

It could take longer (7)

Figure 7.4 Strength of driving and restraining forces

The final stage of the analysis is to develop an action plan which reduces or redirects the restraining forces. Alternatively, action could be geared to increasing the driving forces, but care must be taken because in the process of increasing one force, another force restraining change might be strengthened. It is rarely possible to address all the restraining forces, but even altering one should tip the balance towards the desired change.

The workshop group that looked at handover of patient care developed an action plan to address the concern over breaching confidentiality. This is given in Figure 7.5. In this instance the action plan is rather general because the participants at the workshop were drawn from different NDUs. If the exercise had been undertaken in one NDU one would expect to see a more carefully targeted action plan, identifying timing, what resources might be needed, what support might be needed and any training required.

Action Plan

To address fear of breaching confidentiality

1. Aim to find a place where handover can be done without being overheard.

2. Training – around issues such as access and control of information. Maybe experiential learning.

3. A working practice that allows patients to say what is confidential to them. This needs training and joint planning.

4. Pilot study to see if patients felt handover by beds breached confidentiality.

Figure 7.5 Confidentiality action plan

The impact of change

Developments in nursing practice, even when these seem to be small changes, can require fundamental alterations in our roles and sometimes in ourselves. Changes in role entail new relationships with our colleagues and in turn impact on all aspects of clinical practice including how we develop strategies for change, leadership and teamwork.

Each person involved in an innovation might ask themselves some questions about what the innovation means to them:

- What does this do to my status in the organisation?
- Will it mean my work is different?
- Will it alter my routines?
- How will it be perceived by others whom I respect outside the immediate work situation?

This sort of analysis can be explicit or implicit (Stocking 1985). The case study in the previous chapter illustrates how even a change which we fully favour can be very unsettling at the personal level. It is much more difficult to bring about change that is incompatible with roles or with professional attitudes. A clear example of this, both in NDUs and outside, is how difficult it has been to alter the patients' day so that they can follow their normal sleeping pattern. Even where nurses change their behaviour, there are the physiotherapists, occupational therapists and a host of others to take into account.

A final consideration, but one which has been extremely important in the King's Fund Centre work, has been the context in which this stage of the NDU work has been undertaken. The first two and a half years of the project saw considerable change in the NHS – the introduction of clinical directorates, the separation of health commissioners or purchasers from providers, and the push for trust status from some provider units. Much of this reorganisation has been accompanied by hyperbole which serves both to increase the excitement of the instigators of change and to raise the anxiety of those who feel powerless to effect the way in which it is happening. Much of the work undertaken with the projects has involved helping nurses to feel less powerless and while maybe not excited by the changes, able to influence them.

Review – formal and informal

The starting and finishing point of any cycle of change is the review process. Both Camberwell and Brighton NDUs had major action research taking place focusing on the activity of the units. The collection, analysis and presentation of data to the staff inevitably formed a major review exercise for the unit. However, such work is laborious and, in the case of Brighton, was not started until six months into the project. In Camberwell, while the data were collected early on in the project, interpretation of the data and presentation to the staff took a long time. Time distanced the staff from the research and created problems of ownership for the staff.

Speedier methods of review were also used. Joy Warren in West Dorset NDU used a research method to help the staff clarify the issues around their implementation of primary nursing. She interviewed as many of the staff as she could using a semi-structured interview schedule, drew from the interviews broad categories which she then presented to the staff in a NDU meeting and made available a written copy of the report. The process was the same as the research process but the style and objectives were similar to the methods of classic consultancy. She telescoped the whole process into a few weeks; the diagnosis stage of consultancy could take just one morning.

In Brighton, a workshop was held to review the progress made in the first year of the project and to identify some goals and priorities for the following year. Although such an event is less formal than research, it requires considerable effort in terms of planning and facilitation to ensure that all staff have the opportunity to participate. In this case, Brenda Hawkey planned the event for a Saturday, when it was possible to use the gym on the floor below the ward. The workshop was divided into a series of small groups on particular topics decided by the team. The staff then opted to attend the small groups that interested them; Brenda juggled the small groups so that staff could attend and the ward was adequately staffed. Other ways of making time that have been employed in NDUs include dividing the team into two so that one half covers for the other half to meet and entering into reciprocal arrangements with other teams, for example with another ward or with a research and development team.

It is vital that a review celebrates the successes of the unit, however small they might be. Quite often in the NDUs staff would bewail their lack of progress or lack of achievement. As an outsider it was sometimes easier for me to see what had been achieved, whereas once staff had developed their practice it was sometimes difficult for them to remember where they had come from; the good practice became a norm and therefore unremarkable. The review also needs to look at the difficult issues, the things that one cannot be proud of, and it is important to handle these in a way that is not accusatory or dispiriting, but allows people to express how they feel and voice their opinions. Ground rules can be helpful in setting the scene so that those participating feel they can speak openly. Good facilitation with attention paid to the three strands of interaction – information, process and emotions – can help people feel safe. Often all that is required is the transfer of the skills and approach we employ for patients to working with our colleagues.

Each NDU produced an annual report at the end of the year. Each pursued its own style but all the reports had the following components:

- How the unit got here – for the first year there needed to be a description of the process of being awarded a grant
- The overall vision for the unit
- What the unit set out to achieve in this particular year
- What the unit did achieve: evaluations, results of any auditing help to flesh out the picture
- What helped and what hindered progress
- Goals for the forthcoming year: these were not necessarily detailed but the key areas for future development work were identified
- Annual accounts for the NDU and projected budget for the forthcoming year

The report was presented to the NDU steering group, which consisted of a wide range of disciplines and, in some cases, lay members. This meant that the report had to be accessible to interested and committed people who did not necessarily have a detailed understanding of nursing issues.

Talking to the nurses in the NDUs, it is apparent that the mechanics of being an NDU get easier as they become more familiar. Having presented to the first steering group, or written your first annual report, the second holds few terrors. Some skill development and discussion with other team members also helps, particularly in building confidence.

Dissemination and spread

Implicit in the NDU approach is a critique of top-down, blanket approaches to change. Many nurses have experienced the negative aspects of this type of change. The NDU approach tolerated and encouraged diversity – small groups of nurses finding their own solutions to nursing problems and evaluating them. Given this basic principle it was not surprising that the NDUs did things differently from other teams of nurses and from each other. The NDU was not a remedial strategy to impose good practice on areas with specific problems; that was for management to solve. It was also likely that where there were already differing standards of care between one unit or team in the same organisation, this might become more pronounced as a team with already good standards of care made a specific effort to develop practice. However, this was a particularly hard nettle to grasp.

Three related issues arose from this aspect of the approach. First, being different was equated both within and outside the units as being elitist. I have no measure of how elitist the units were thought to be by their colleagues, but some of the nurses in the units and some of their managers believed that that was how they were perceived. As a consequence some managers tended to minimise the achievements of the NDU within the organisation and the staff in the units retreated rather than promoted themselves. Inadvertently, we at the King's Fund contributed to that retreat by suggesting that the units should be 'protected areas' for the first year to enable them to develop without publicity. Thinking back to that time, I wonder how much we were protecting the units and how much we were protecting ourselves – taking risks was difficult for us as well.

Reversing that approach and developing effective communication strategies for each unit was extremely hard, despite excellent consultancy from Lynne Woodward, director of communications at the King's Fund Centre. Early initiatives to promote the individual units within their organisations were often reactive – to resell the idea of an NDU to a new management team – rather than to tell other nurses about developments and what nurses in the units were learning about change.

The third thorny area that arose from the principle that teams of nurses should be allowed to develop their own initiatives was the issue of spread. We at the Nursing Developments Programme and many of the managers supporting the units recognised that progress would be made if the project remained focused around a strong team, with other nurses outside the unit making their own decisions as to which innovations to adopt or whether they should investigate alternative ways of tackling the same issue. However, this was contrary to the prevalent culture of the NHS, where change would be 'rolled out' or 'cascaded down'. I had one discussion with a chief executive in which in his efforts to adopt the flattened principle of the NDU he exhorted me to get the programme 'cascaded out'.

As the project progressed and the NDUs became more established, alternatives to geographical spread, planned and unplanned, in which an NDU can influence an organisation became evident:

- In some organisations there was competition from other wards and teams. This may have been uncomfortable for the NDUs

concerned and uncomfortable for the wards involved, but like the grit in the oyster it overall produced a bigger pearl.
- Various planned outreach activities occurred, often with a member of the NDU giving dedicated consultancy time to assist other individuals and teams. In some instances this required careful negotiation to ensure that these activities did not erode impetus in the NDU.

The ways and means of development work

Each of the four NDUs went through a planned change process. Part of the development work was to make that process explicit and shared throughout the team. All the units started with a vision of how they would like to develop nursing over the next three years. As the project progressed, NDU staff worked on developing realisable objectives, working out who were the best people to lead the work and allocating time and support to those piloting developments and reviewing and evaluating their progress.

As well as a planned cycle, we at the King's Fund Centre and staff in the units were able to look at new ways of influencing the cycle of change. We paid particular attention to the three strands of interaction: to technical content, to the way the process happens and to the underlying currents of emotion. Particularly important was how change, even change that is fully supported, makes the people involved feel.

Second, staff in the NDUs found it was necessary to use their management skills with those higher up the organisation as well as those they managed; this was an essential component of leadership. In the context of major organisational change in the NHS, an appreciation of how the senior managers were experiencing those changes was important in working with them on nursing development.

When it was difficult to know how to bring about a change or things seemed to have got stuck, continuing to push the required change is often counterproductive and it is more useful to look at how to reduce the things that are preventing the change from happening (the restraining forces).

Finally, nurses set themselves very high standards and even when they make considerable progress and innovation, they tend to look for what they are not doing rather than what has been achieved. We all worked to foster an environment which celebrated achievement and looked for support and help when things did not go well. In this we were all helped by the willingness of others in the 'family of nursing' who were willing to share our vision.

References

Gabbaro J and Kotter J (1980) Managing your boss. *Harvard Business Review*, January-February.

Lewin K (1951) *Field Theory in Social Science*. London: Harper & Row.

Stocking B (1985) *Initiative and Inertia: Case Studies in the NHS*. London: Nuffield Provincial Hospitals Trust.

CHAPTER 8

NDUs and Nursing Knowledge and Education

Barbara Vaughan

Over the past decade there has been a growing interest in exactly what it is that constitutes 'nursing knowledge' and more importantly what knowledge expert practitioners call on in order to be able to nurse effectively. Nursing development units have been contributing to the exploration of nursing knowledge – by developing nurses themselves and testing the nature and practice of nursing. This chapter will explore some of the implications of the expansion of nursing knowledge as undertaken in NDUs.

In many ways it is curious that it has taken us, as nurses, so long to wake up to the fact that we have very limited understanding or formal theory about the practice of nursing as a whole, nor about the nature of the knowledge we draw on in making clinical judgements. Much of the skill of day-to-day practice has remained hidden and unacknowledged, often devalued as 'ordinary' or 'commonplace', and greater emphasis has been placed on that which can be gleaned from the textbook than from that which can be gleaned from practice itself. Lawler (1991) suggests that 'the essence of these practices [clinical nursing] has not been deemed as formal knowledge, partly because there has been no formal language to describe them'. Thus little attention has been paid to trying to gain a greater understanding of the way in which the fundamental work of nurses, which is inextricably concerned with care, can play a part in healing. It has been suggested that this has led, over a period of time, to nursing work becoming invisible in terms of its impact on health gain, the argument being that:

> the 'invisibility' of nursing is linked with these concepts (body care, privacy, dirty work, etc.) and with the lack of an academic discourse on the body as a *whole*. (Lawler 1991)

Yet there is no doubt that expert decision-making goes on all the time in the clinical setting albeit from a knowledge base which is often 'tacit' or hidden. In many ways it is the clinical setting which is our 'laboratory' for enquiry, not only as a site for exploring new issues in nursing, but also as a site in which students can learn.

Nursing development units

In some ways NDUs can be seen as laboratories of this kind, offering an environment where scholarly enquiry, research and learning are part of everyday practice. By their very nature they foster a climate where old ideas can be tested and challenged and new ideas can be formulated and, in their turn, evaluated. Questioning becomes the norm and change is commonplace. Thus, in relationship to both nurse education and the further development of nursing knowledge it is the context that NDUs provide which is so critical.

While it can be argued that nurse education and the development of nursing knowledge are inextricably linked, for convenience they will be discussed separately in this chapter. However, it is the very 'wholeness' of NDUs, where all these activities are fostered within the same environment, which makes them stand out as different. It is important not to lose sight of this idea throughout.

Nursing knowledge

In order to grasp the way in which NDUs can contribute to the development of nursing knowledge it is necessary first to take a brief look at the things that have influenced nursing research over the years. As nurses have striven to seek scientific recognition of their work many have been influenced by the research methods which have been dominant in other related disciplines, predominantly in medicine and psychology. Thus they have been lured into a *positivist* world where there is a basic belief that everything that is worth knowing can be reduced to that which is visible and measurable (Hammersley and Atkinson 1983). Cause and effect relationships have been sought between nursing practice and patient outcomes, an admirable and essential purpose in professional, economic and political terms. In many ways the purpose behind such work has been to provide a degree of certainty about the types of practice which will produce the best results and much valuable knowledge has been gained in this way.

Essentially, the driving force behind work of this nature has been the desire to collate objective evidence of the world of nursing. What was seen as critical was the researcher's ability to remain distanced from the subject of enquiry, whether patients or nurses, putting to one side feelings or personal values which may bias the results. Thus it was necessary for those who undertook research in nursing to be separate from those who were the subjects of enquiry – that is, the practising nurses themselves. This reductionist approach can be seen today in the way in which nursing work roles have developed, with a sharp divide between those who practise, teach, manage or research. However, NDUs provide an environment where new unified roles, such as that of the joint appointee (Wright 1989), the lecturer/manager practitioner (Vaughan 1990) or the primary nurse/project worker (Garbett 1992) can be explored and developed.

In the same vein, great importance has been placed in the past on drawing knowledge from other disciplines and attempting to apply it deductively to nursing. There has been an emphasis on using the knowledge of physiologists, psychologists, sociologists and many others in nursing work. However, as Street (1990) points out:

> Even in the professions least equipped with a secure foundation of systematic professional knowledge . . . yearning for the rigour of science-based knowledge and the power of science-based techniques leads schools to import scholars from neighbouring departments of social sciences.

Maybe it is the very fact that nursing research and nursing practice have been separated that has led to such a situation. While the knowledge gained in this way has been of value, it can be suggested that such distancing has also led to a lack of enquiry about the unique knowledge of nursing practice itself. Street (1990) argues that 'the positivist paradigm which endorses the view that practice is developed by the application of knowledge remains dominant.' In her view it is the introduction of such a wide range of subjects in nurse education that has hoodwinked nurses into believing that this gives academic respectability, while in reality nursing programmes

> may appear to be providing a different pair of lenses for viewing and understanding practice – in reality the same image is being broadened and deepened without changing the essential elements: that is the images and values of the positivist paradigm are being endorsed.

Further reasons why such a situation has arisen are obscure, but may be partly attributed to a lack of understanding of the complexity of many nursing acts or because, by their very nature, they are 'private', leading to a lack of willingness on the part of both nurses and others to discuss and explore them openly.

While objectivity has its place to play in nursing enquiry, there has been a growing interest in the interpersonal nature of much that occurs in practice. Since nursing and people cannot be separated, it has gradually been recognised that the traditional scientific approach, which separates researcher and subject, can only give us answers to one small part of the total world of practice from either the patients' or the nurses' perspective. Indeed, the Audit Commission (1992) suggests that it is very difficult to make cause and effect relationships between nursing care and patient outcomes because of the wide range of variables which may influence any individual's progress.

In line with this recognition there has been a need to look to alternative research methods, with a movement away from the distanced objective scientist to a researcher who becomes immersed in the real world of practice and attempts to interpret that world as it is perceived by those within it. Such approaches are commonly concerned with the meaning of phenomena, such as loss, motivation or caring, as they are experienced by the patients or clients themselves. This interpretative approach draws on qualitative research methods such as ethnography or phenomenology, as a means of helping us to understand how the world is seen by others, recognising that not everyone places the same meaning on the same experience.

One of the significant features of this shift is the change of emphasis in the relationship between the researcher and the subject. If meanings are important, then immersion in the subjects' world also becomes important, and it can be argued that NDUs are an ideal site for such work to be carried out. While expert practice is by no means exclusive to NDUs, they do provide a setting where the staff have learned to be more articulate about both positive and worrying aspects of their work and by their very nature many of them have been involved in some form of continuing education. It is not necessarily the fact that they are practising with more expertise than others which makes them so suitable for such enquiry. This would be an unreal expectation. Rather, it is that they have gained experience in expressing what it is that they do and thus are able to open up areas of their practice more readily for scrutiny by both themselves and others.

The final step in this movement along the continuum of approaches to research takes us into the realms of critical social theory (Smythe 1986), where there is a greater emphasis on the growth or emancipation of the person (in this case both the nurse and the patient) as a means of empowerment. While these are strong words, the basic argument is that unless people see themselves as free to act, then much of the knowledge they have lies hidden and dormant. It is only when they take ownership of themselves and the world in which they live that they are able to develop their practice. How often do we, as nurses, hear ourselves saying: 'But am I allowed to . . .?' One of the exciting things about NDUs is that the question shifts from 'Am I allowed to . . .?' to 'What would be gained (by nurses and patients) if . . .?' This does not mean that there is an open door for anyone to do anything, since we are all constrained to a greater or lesser extent by many factors in the world in which we live. What it does imply is an attitudinal change from one of perceived helplessness to one of perceived power. Provided that power to ask questions and to act on hunches is used positively, this can be one of the richest sources in the development of nursing knowledge.

The most commonly used method of enquiry in the realms of critical social theory is that of action research (Carr and Kemmis 1984), which provides a cyclical approach to identifying problems as perceived by the people themselves, helping them to find local solutions which will bring about change. As its name implies, it is an action-oriented method, which involves everyone as equal partners in the scene. Furthermore, it is based on a model of empowerment which closely reflects the value systems of many people working within NDUs. The emancipatory knowledge gained in this way is primarily concerned with the ability to 'act rationally, to reason self-consciously and to make decisions on the basis of available knowledge and need' (Pearson 1992).

Turning back to NDUs as sites where nursing knowledge may be developed, they can potentially be a rich site for generating questions in all three domains which have been described. Indeed, the responsibility of those who work in NDUs goes beyond the point of striving to seek excellence in practice to the point of challenging norms and questioning many traditional practices. A critical feature of an NDU is the creation of an environment where enquiry, change, challenge and development are a part of everyday life. However, it must be added that this is not always an easy world to live in and takes considerable courage and strength on the part of the practitioners. Without emancipatory knowledge, some may find it too difficult to survive in such a challenging setting. Yet if norms are not challenged, there would be no progress and development would be stifled.

Each of the approaches to exploring nursing knowledge has a value and it is important that respect is given to the whole range of methods of exploration. For example, both Pearson et al (1992) and Sleep (1991) used randomised controlled trials, which are within the positivist school, the former to look at the use of nursing beds and the latter to assess the value of episiotomy. Benner (1984) used a phenomenological approach in her exploration of expert practice; more recently Morrison (1992) studied caring within this framework which is interpretative. Action research is also gaining popularity with nurses and has been used, among others, by Webb (1991), Titchen and Binnie (1992) and all who were facilitating the development of different aspects of practice.

Challenging norms

It is difficult to be precise about the types of enquiry which occur in NDUs as many of them arise out of the experiences of practice itself. There are, however, two basic approaches. First, there is a need to explore the use of ideas which may have been developed elsewhere. However, in many instances ideas need adjusting and modifying to meet the local needs of both the client group and the organisation. For example, self-medication has been explored by many nurses over the last few years and there is considerable evidence that it can have an impact on patients' understanding of the way in which the drugs they are taking work, the times at which they should be taken and the potential problematic side-effects which may occur (e.g. Bird 1990). However, the manner in which this practice is brought into being in different settings is dependent on many local circumstances, such as the service which pharmacists can supply, the facilities for storage of drugs, the knowledge of the nurses who will be involved in helping patients to learn about their medication, the resistance of some colleagues in other disciplines and the particular clinical needs of the patient group. Thus it is not a case simply of taking the work of others and rigidly applying it locally, as would occur within the positivist paradigm, but of taking the basic principles of the idea and modifying them to meet local need. There can be two outcomes from work of this kind. First, our understanding of the efficacy and potential hazards of the practice can be deepened as the experiences of a wider range of practitioners and patients are explored. Second, from the work of the nurses on the NDU, local policies and learning programmes can be developed for other nurses working in similar situations as well as providing a demonstration site.

The second area of enquiry which arises out of NDUs is when they seek to gain an increased understanding of a particular area of practice which has not been explored in depth elsewhere. One example of work of this kind was that of Pearson et al (1992) in relation to the use of nursing beds. Other areas which have been or are being explored include such things as increasing the opportunity for patients to have more choice and control in their own care, the impact of continuity of care on patient outcomes, the way in which motivation for recovery can influence the rate and way in which patients regain optimal health and the impact of nursing clinics on patient outcomes. The areas are endless but it would be inappropriate to pre-empt them all here as the very nature of an NDU indicates that they arise out of practice rather than are imposed on it. This does not mean that they are not transferable in principle, but that the responsibility for raising questions lies with the practitioners rather than from an outside source.

NDUs as sites for learning

Since nursing is a practice discipline, the most critical responsibility we have towards nurse learners and those involved in continuing education is to provide opportunities for them to develop their skills in practice. There is undoubtedly a huge backdrop of formal knowledge which can be explored theoretically, through the literature and other study methods, within the safety of an academic institute. However, there is a critical difference between that which can be learned from textbooks and the ability which people need to make use of, and sometimes transform, that knowledge in practice. It is in learning to make use of knowledge in practice that NDUs have such a critical role to play. Smythe (1986) suggests that much of what is presented as truth or fact within a scientific framework is fine in 'the high moral ground . . . of research-based theory for seeking resolutions to out problems.' But he goes on to suggest that there are times when this type of work becomes incompatible and discredited when we 'descend into the swampy lowlands where situations are murky and characterised by confusing messes with no easy resolution.'

How easily this situation can be recognised in nursing, where the procedure book or textbook may tell us how things should be done, but takes no account of many of the contextual demands of reality such as lack of equipment, the individuality of patients or an 'intuitive' knowledge that this is the one patient among many others who does *not* want to know what will be happening and would prefer to be told what is best. Drawing on the work of Benner (1984), novice practitioners lean heavily on the formal theory they have been taught to make clinical decisions, whereas observation of expert practitioners shows how they have moved on from the need to rely on formal procedures. In some circumstance Schon (1987) suggests that the experts are 'surprised' by some observation which helps them to recognise that this situation does not fit the textbook pattern. They then draw on the whole background of their knowledge, often at a subconscious level, which has been gained through both formal study and experience, to make judgements and take actions which are unique to the individual situation. This 'wisdom, artistry or intuition' in practice has not, in the past, been deemed to be academically respectable. However, within the environment of an NDU exploration of intuitive practices is encouraged rather than dismissed and this exploration may in its turn lead to a *transformation* of some of our understanding of nursing knowledge.

The question which this raises is how we can help the novice practitioners to move towards such expert practice. This is where NDUs have an important part to play. There is no doubt that time and experience are needed for this transition to occur. However, there are also strategies which can be brought into play which can facilitate the transition and help people to move from a position of dependence on rule-based practice to one of perceived freedom where autonomous judgements, which sometimes seem to defy usual practice, can be made.

Reflection in action

One strategy which has come into prominence in recent times is the use of 'reflection in action' and 'reflection on action', heavily influenced by the work of Schon (1987), as a means of unravelling the chaos of the world of practice. This is an approach which many practitioners within NDUs and other settings are starting to use as a means of learning to survive and become creative in the so-called 'swampy lowlands'. Schon argues that students cannot be taught to 'use' rather than 'apply' knowledge. Thus it is not possible to 'teach' people the vast area of factors which may impinge on a clinical decision. They can, however, be 'coached' and, in exploring through reflection what they have seen with their own eyes, start to make sense of reality.

Reflection in action has become a very popular term and there is no doubt that it can be an extremely valuable approach in helping students and experienced practitioners alike to deepen their understanding of practice (or indeed other aspects of their role such as teaching or managing). Reflective journals are one way in which active reflection can be enhanced. Indeed, this is a practice which is not uncommon among NDU staff themselves. It is important, however, to be quite clear that there is a critical difference between keeping a diary and keeping a reflective journal. Reflective journals go well beyond a record of events to a critical and personal analysis of the experience for the writer. They offer the opportunity to explore what meaning an incident had, what formal and intuitive knowledge was used and potentially what gaps were present in that person's understanding of what happened, as a person and as a nurse. They are intensely personal in nature, with ownership firmly vested in the person who makes the recording, and there must be choice in what is and what is not revealed. In this way it is possible to be open and honest with oneself, whereas, if there is foreknowledge that the journal would be scrutinised by others, there may be caution in the way recordings are made (Vaughan 1992).

However, much of what is gained by keeping a reflective journal would be lost if some of the experiences were not shared. Furthermore, the pressure of self-exploration could become intense if there were not an opportunity to explore with others some of the understanding which may arise out of the experience of reflection. Peer groups or team meetings may be used to facilitate sharing, clinical supervision or mentorship systems can be established where partners are chosen or people external to the situation may help to develop the skills needed. In many NDUs this is a chosen method which has been used to help the nurses gain group cohesion, come to understand their practice more fully and identify areas which they feel need further development through review of the literature, seeking expert help or more formal research.

Keeping a journal is not the only way in which reflection can be encouraged. Schon (1987) recommends working with a 'coach' who can help people to identify strengths in their own work, which may otherwise go unacknowledged, as well as exploring learning needs. A coach, however, is very different from the clinical teacher, who may teach someone how to practise. The coach works through the learner's own experience or acts as a role model, helping the learner to gain insight into his or her own actions. As a word of warning it should be added here that there is grave doubt about whether someone can facilitate reflection in either of these ways, unless that person has *personal* experience of reflection.

Links with others

By the nature of their work those who practise in NDUs often keep journals for themselves as well as acting as coaches to new team members and others. Journal writing may, however, also offer a way in which links can be made with those who are based in more formal educational settings. An NDU can offer a 'safe haven' for teachers who need time to develop their own understanding of practice and reflect on that experience (Gray and Forsstrom 1992). In turn, there are many skills, such as a more formal insight into nursing theory, maybe a deeper knowledge of nursing literature and experience of research skills, which a teacher will have developed, but may not be common to all NDU staff. The relationship between an NDU and an educational department is collegial in nature with both parties respecting each other's work. Reciprocity is a feature which has been identified as important in nurse–patient relationships (Cahill 1991), but is of equal importance in sharing knowledge and experience between practitioners and teachers. Thus those working in education are in a position to help the NDU staff to extend their skills in one way while those in the NDU can help the teachers to develop in another.

For teachers, an NDU may be the site they can go to to gain experience of using model-based assessment and coming to understand the strengths and weaknesses of different approaches to care. It may be the site where they gather knowledge through experience, which, in turn, they can use to make sense of their own teaching, both for themselves and for the students.

NDUs can also act as a site for role–modelling for the students. While the NDU staff, by their very nature, may not have 'applied' theory in its literal form they will certainly have used it to inform their actions. In turn, teachers may have access to experience of writing, of running workshops or conferences or of preparing materials which may help the NDU staff to develop teaching programmes for the patients or clients. Help may also be forthcoming in preparing publicity material about the unit. Since dissemination of their work is a fundamental feature of an NDU, this can be a vital resource.

Thus the nature of the relationship between educational settings and NDUs is one of mutual support and sharing, a partnership where each has something to offer the other. The opportunity to test and, if need be, transform theory is an expected norm, as is the generation of new ideas and exploration of alternative practices.

Conclusion

The perpetual need nurses have to go on seeking new knowledge as a means of improving practice is a demanding but exciting challenge. Bringing together those who work in NDUs and those who work in nurse education can act as a powerful force in helping to meet this end. There is a mutual goal of all nurses concerned with improving patient care, and this can only be achieved by deepening our understanding of the way in which nursing can promote health and healing. Through a cyclical process practitioners and teachers can be nurtured and nourished by each other's experiences and insights, with mutual respect gained for all the contributions which can be made towards developing practice.

Nursing is at an exciting stage in its development and there is a growing recognition of the contribution which we, as nurses, can make to health care. Those who work in NDUs have an important part to play in gaining further insight into this contribution. Similarly, it is the teachers who have the responsibility of guiding learning for both new and experienced nurses, alongside the expertise in analysis and interpretation of theory. Each in its own way contributes to the future of nursing. Together, they are a powerful force for improving patient care.

References

Audit Commission (1992) *Making Time for Patients: A Handbook for Ward Sisters*. London: HMSO.

Benner P (1984) *From Novice to Expert – Excellence and Power in Clinical Nursing Practice*. Menlo Park, CA: Addison-Wesley.

Bird C (1990) Drug administration: A prescription for self-help. *Nursing Times* **86**(43): 52–55.

Cahill M (1991) *Effective Nursing – An Exploration by Experienced Nurses*. Oxford: Ashdale Press.

Carr W and Kemmis S (1984) *Becoming Critical – Knowing Through Action Research*. Geelong, Victoria: Deakin University Press.

Garbett R (1992) Nursing development units – attested development. *Nursing Times* **88**(35): 40–42.

Gray J and Forsstrom S (1992) Generating Theory from Practice: The Reflective Technique. In J Gray and R Pratt, *Towards a Discipline of Nursing*. London: Churchill Livingstone.

Hammersley M and Atkinson P (1983) *Ethnography – Principles in Practice.* Cambridge: Cambridge University Press.

Lawler J (1991) *Behind the Screens.* London: Churchill Livingstone.

Morrison P (1992) *Professional Caring in Practice: A Psychological Analysis.* Aldershot: Avebury.

Pearson A (1992) *Nursing at Burford – A Story of Change.* London: Scutari Press.

Pearson A, Punton S and Durand I (1992) *Nursing Beds: An Evaluation of the Effects of Therapeutic Nursing.* London: Scutari Press.

Schon D (1987) *Educating the Reflective Practitioner.* Oxford: Jossey-Bass.

Sleep J (1991) Perineal Care: A Series of Five Randomised Controlled Trials. In S Robinson and A Thompson (eds) *Midwives, Research and Childbirth,* vol 2. London: Chapman & Hall.

Smythe W J (1986) *Reflection in Action.* Geelong, Victoria: Deakin University Press.

Street A (1990) *Nursing Practice: High, Hard Ground, Messy Swamps and Pathways in Between.* Geelong, Victoria: Deakin University Press.

Titchen A and Binnie A (1992) *A Unified Action Research Strategy in Nursing.* Unpublished paper. Oxford: Institute of Nursing.

Vaughan B (1990) The Role of the Lecturer Practitioner. In J Salvage and B Kershaw (eds) *Models for Nursing,* vol 2. London: Scutari Press.

Vaughan B (1992) Exploring the Knowledge of Nursing Practice. *Journal of Clinical Nursing* **1**: 161–166.

Webb C (1991) Action research: philosophy, methods and personal experiences. *Journal of Advanced Nursing* **14**(5): 403–410.

Wright S (1989) *An Evaluation of Joint Appointments in Nursing.* Department of Life Sciences: Huddersfield Polytechnic.

CHAPTER 9

Evaluating Nursing

Rebecca Malby

'No one understands us. We're not paid enough for what we do. We're expected to do more with less. We're not valued, we're treated like skivvies.' This is a common theme for nurses, be it chatting over coffee, at sisters' meetings, at conference question times or in the opinion columns of the press. How often do we try to advance as a profession, only to find that there are not the resources and/or the commitment by our colleagues – nurses, doctors or managers – to support us. Then we blame others, labelling them as the 'opposition', adopting the roles of victim and heroine, the saviours of caring in an uncaring service. We also protest, waving the flags of standards of care and patient advocacy to show how right we are. So where does it all go wrong? Can it really be that the 'opposition' are out to trample us underfoot with an army of health care assistants?

The meteoric rise of NDUs seems to show that it is possible to develop nursing practice in an environment where the nurse's contribution to the team is valued and where nurses act in partnership with patients and other professionals to determine care. So what is the key to success that turns nurses as victims into nurses as leaders and enables other professionals to start thinking of nurses as a vital component in the delivery of the service? Part of that success lies in evaluation: that recognises all professionals' concerns about the service and the language they speak and that empowers nurses to choose the best practice for their patients.

When nurses say they have evaluated a new pressure-relieving mattress and found that it improves the quality of care, and that they would like £10000 to buy mattresses for the hospital, the manager's thinking may go like this: 'That's X amount of theatre time, which means Y fewer patients treated, which means that

Mr Bloggs will have to wait Z more months for his hip operation, which means that I will get five more letters from his MP and there will be another question in the House, which means that I will have to cancel all cataract surgery in order to get Mr Bloggs his operation.' However, the nurse might say to the manager: 'We have evaluated this mattress and have found that although it costs £100, it reduces the incidence of pressure sores by X per cent. Our current incidence of pressure sores is Y. The average cost of a pressure sore is £Z (consisting of nursing time, dressings, increased length of stay and medication). If we had enough mattresses for the hospital we would save (X/100 x Y) x (Z minus £100) x number required, minus training costs of £A.' Then the manager will think: 'That will help me get Mr Bloggs in for his operation X months early, so I can get four more off the waiting list, which means that the Community Health Council will be happy, Mr Surgeon will be happy and the MP will stop pestering us.'

We have evaluated the mattress, recognising that the manager's job is to make the best use of the money available. From our point of view we may be evaluating the mattress for patient comfort, ability to help prevent pressure sores, impact on cross-infection, ability to be cleaned, ease of use and cost. All of these are valid in terms of the quality of care and important in reviewing the best support to our practice. The manager should be clear that in our professional judgement this is the best value for money, but he or she will be concerned about whether it is the best use of resources. The nurse can recognise the manager's concerns and describe the outcome of the evaluation in a language that addresses those concerns and achieves the results she wanted.

Evaluation in an NDU

An NDU is a laboratory for the organisation and practice of nursing, so it must demonstrate the fruits of its work. It needs to identify which models of professional practice offer the best care and the best value for money. It also needs to establish a process of review to enable practitioners to plan the way forward for nursing, empowering the staff to choose the direction of the NDU. Some of the concerns that need to be addressed are related to the agendas of the various groups interested in the outcomes of the health service. These include the following:

- *Consumer (or patient) agenda.* The public is demanding more choice and therefore more information. The rise of individualism in the Thatcher era has introduced a new focus on the 'consumer' throughout the public sector. However, while consumers still rely on representatives to purchase their care (such as GPs or purchasing consortia), pressure groups and consumer lobbies are calling for patient participation and information. This goes hand in hand with the philosophy of an NDU which seeks to empower patients through empowered staff. If the role of an NDU is to provide the best for patients, then patient concerns must be pivotal to any evaluation.

- *Political and policy agenda.* Social policy over the last decade has highlighted evaluation, particularly in the areas of assessment of performance (Pollitt 1986) and value for money. Roberts (1991) says the reasons for being interested in the performance of the health service are clear: 'to establish in aggregate whether we are getting value for expenditure on health services and whether those services are effective.' One such initiative in the NHS has been the development of performance indicators (clinical, managerial, financial and estate management) to be used in the new culture of managerial accountability (Pollitt 1984). These indicators were a response to the belief that productivity could be increased through improved performance, according to financial expediency. Another initiative was the focus on resource management, involving clinicians in management to make them more accountable for the resources they commit. The quest for performance measurement materialised in the Government White Paper 'Working for Patients', in the form of medical audit and the introduction of the internal health care market. Nursing is all too easily marginalised from these initiatives: this was so in resource management (Packwood et al 1991) and in medical audit. Nurses must become involved in nursing and clinical (multidisciplinary) audit as a means of evaluation and assessment of care (Hancock 1990, Salvage 1990). NDUs can capitalise on this interest in evaluation, particularly in the form of audit.
- *Managerial agenda.* The managerial agenda is closely linked to the political agenda and achieving value for money. In the new NHS this translates into the language of contracts, which specify cost, quality and volume. NDUs must determine the effect on the contracting process of developments in the organisation and practice of nursing. Having an NDU in a provider unit which evaluates the influence of the nursing contribution on the cost, quality and volume of contracts while seeking to achieve excellence may be a selling point for

managers seeking service developments through new contracts. It will also enable them to predict the effect of developments in nursing on the service as a whole. All this must be done in a managerial climate that assesses critically the number of qualified nurses required and the nature of the support roles. Thus NDUs may be at the forefront of evaluating the impact of empowered, autonomous nurses on contracting.

- *Professional agenda*. The need to develop nursing practice has been discussed in previous chapters. To do this, nurses must be able to assess new and current practices to determine what is best. This evaluation enables nurses to develop their roles and to become critical and analytical, rejecting routine for routine's sake. It enables nurses to make choices rather than be dictated to by years of tradition. Doing it sister's way because sister says so will become a thing of the past. Doing it my way, because my patient and I judge that to be the best way, is the hope of the future. Nursing is striving for more autonomous practice (Pearson et al 1989) and for partnership with other health care professionals (particularly doctors) in decision-making about patient care (Stein et al 1990).

Evaluation literally means assessing value. It is therefore strongly linked with the values of NDUs, which in turn are linked with the values of the profession: values such as patient and carer involvement in care, partnership and sharing, models of health rather than disease and human rights to confidentiality and choice. There are several approaches to evaluation. These include evaluation of the following: a particular change in practice (e.g. changing from fixed shifts to flexitime); current practices to choose the best for your own situation (e.g. primary versus team nursing, or one dressing versus another); the evaluation of the NDU in relation to one of the agendas above (e.g. using a yearly audit); and the impact of the NDU on nursing in other areas (wards, clinics, community teams) in the unit (community, acute). There are many types of evaluation, each with an associated method of collecting information, so it is important to determine the aims of the evaluation – to determine the best dressing for a leg ulcer, to make the case for additional resources, to explore the contribution of the qualified nurse, to assess the importance of the NDU, or to find out what areas of the nursing service require development.

Evaluating an NDU

The most crucial point to note in evaluating an NDU is that you must begin at the beginning with some form of baseline measurement. You can then evaluate the current situation and in future evaluate the impact of the NDU in relation to those baseline measurements. This enables you to make 'before and after' studies. If you do not know the features of clinical area before you start making changes, how will you know whether you are making progress?

It is likely that you will want to evaluate the impact of the NDU on the quality of care, efficiency and effectiveness (given the prevailing political and managerial agendas). This takes time! It is important to make time both to familiarise yourselves with the literature and to plan how you are going to tackle the audit. At the outset it is difficult to decide what data to collect, but if you have determined the aim of the evaluation, you will have identified the broad categories. Resources, preference and available expertise will dictate whether you use an existing package such as QUALPACS or MONITOR to design your own. If you decide to design your own, advice from a researcher is essential. It is a waste of time to design and distribute a questionnaire only to find that your returns are not a statistically valid sample, thus making your assumptions open to question and your future comparisons invalid. Finally, use what is available. It is likely, for instance, that the administrators collect details of patient throughput, readmissions, staffing costs, cross-infection rates and the dependency or workload. All this is useful for scrutinising current practices and for comparisons in the future. You may find that, over a year, you have significantly reduced the length of time the patient is in contact with the service, or that you reduce the cross-infection rate, or that you reduce staffing costs, or that the workload rises dramatically – all this without having to collect any data, but only drawing conclusions from available information. It is always tempting to collect data on anything that moves, because you don't want to miss anything, but be realistic; there is only so much you can change, so choose what to measure depending on the aims of your evaluation and the timespan between evaluations.

Most NDUs now undertake some form of annual report. This should indicate your evaluation of the progress of the NDU. Thus the minimum frequency for evaluating the NDU should be yearly. This will give you time to plan any changes prompted by your evaluation and to implement them before the next one. Over the year you may want to undertake some spot-checks of progress. If you want a more detailed evaluation of one aspect of the NDU, you could do it as a 'before and after' study, with more detailed data collection.

The key to the success of evaluation is a concept familiar to an NDU: that is decision-making by the whole team. Thus it is important that the NDU team decides the aims of the evaluation, taking into consideration any contractual requirements of the clinical leader of the NDU. Once the data are collected and presented as information, the team will make decisions based on that information, agreeing between themselves the plan of action for change. Then the team is ready to present the information, including the plan, in a form with which they feel comfortable, to their manager. There is a skill in making such a presentation positive, rather than ridden with guilt! Look for the positive outcomes of the evaluation.

Collecting the data is the research phase of the evaluation. In evaluating the NDU as a whole you are likely to want to collect information about a variety of issues (e.g. patient satisfaction, quality of clinical care, workload, costs) and you will need to use a variety of research methods. This may be called a case study, an 'umbrella term for a family of research methods having in common the decision to focus an inquiry round an instance' (Adelman et al 1984). In this case the 'instance' is the NDU. The role of the case study is to explain, illuminate, describe and explore (Yin 1984). Research methods are both qualitative and quantitative. Qualitative research provides the soft, descriptive data, e.g observation (participant and non-participant) or interviews with small, purposive sample sizes. Quantitative research produces the hard data, such as numerical facts, with much larger sample sizes. You may want to use a combination of the two types of research to enable you to evaluate your NDU comprehensively.

An example of a case study

This study used nursing audit to evaluate and plan the developments for an NDU on a surgical ward in a district general hospital. The data collection and interpretation phase of the evaluation took approximately a month, starting from scratch. The audit was designed with reference to other work in this area and recognised the different agendas. Thus the consumer agenda was addressed by using a patient satisfaction interview; the doctors' agenda by using their medical audit results and patient throughput; the managerial agenda by measuring the costs of staffing, sickness and absenteeism and bed occupancy; and the nurses' agenda by using a staff satisfaction questionnaire, monitoring nursing records and measuring patient workload. (Of course, the different agendas overlap and this is a rather simplistic interpretation.) The audit was undertaken in the early days of the NDU and again a year later. The first audit results were used to plan the developments for the first year. The second audit commented on the impact of these developments and was used to plan the following year. The audit was carried out by the nursing development officer (the change agent post).

The method

Patient satisfaction

Patient interviews

A patient interview schedule was designed to elicit patients' views about their nursing care on the ward. The schedule was semi-structured and designed to cover the interviewees' inpatient stay and their preparation for discharge. The design enabled patients to volunteer factual information to enable them to gain confidence before moving on to their perceptions about their care, probed in the interview. The schedule was piloted on the secretaries in the administration department to ensure the neutrality of the questions and ease of comprehension. It was decided to undertake these interviews after the patient had been discharged and before his or her first outpatient appointment, to ensure that the last hospital experience was of the ward and to assess the effectiveness of the discharge. The interviews were conducted by telephone.

The NDU was sometimes used by all specialities in the hospital when their own beds had been filled and there were emergency cases requiring admission. Therefore, the patients to be interviewed were identified as those under the care of the NDU's own consultants. This information was obtained from the patient admission records on the ward. The sample was collected from patients who had been discharged in the month prior to the commencement of the study. Only 75 per cent of the total identified had medical and nursing records available. From these records, clients who had subsequently died, had left the country or had made a formal complaint to the health authority were deselected. Of those remaining, 20 were randomly selected using their personal index number. This amounted to a third of the total number of surgical patients discharged by the ward's consultants in that month. A letter was sent out to those selected so that they would know when to expect the telephone call.

Complaints

Patient complaints are a widely used indicator of patient satisfaction. Therefore the study included the number of written complaints received about the ward and the nature of those complaints. It was noted that complaints can be a positive indicator of nursing, as it means that patients feel they are able to complain.

Nursing staff satisfaction

Staff questionnaire

There are a variety of studies of staff satisfaction and many questionnaires were reviewed. That developed by Humphries and Turner (1989) was chosen as the most suitable. It covered working conditions, emotional climate and general satisfaction, but required some modification to clarify certain points; to add pertinent issues that had arisen since its design (namely clinical grading, which has dramatically affected nurses' pay and their views about their value); to enable nurses to prioritise specific areas of satisfaction and dissatisfaction; and to allow comments. To gain cooperation, the anonymity of the respondent was ensured and explained in the covering instructions for completion of the questionnaire. All the nurses working on the ward, except students, were given the questionnaire with a deadline for completion of two weeks. The nurses were sent a letter reminding them to return the questionnaire three days before the deadline. The completed questionnaires were collected from the letter tray on the deadline day and during the following week.

Sickness and absenteeism

The amount in days of staff sickness and of staff absenteeism per month was collected retrospectively from ward records for a period of three months before the study began. Any periods of sickness of a week or over (i.e. certificated sickness) was noted as a percentage of the whole. The assumption is that staff who have low morale, lack motivation and/or who are stressed will take more unscheduled days off or will absent themselves from work (Patchen 1970).

Clinical indicators

The doctors collect details of post-operative complications for all their patients for their own audit. Those complications that could have been affected by nursing care were selected: chest infections, deep vein thrombosis and wound infections. The incidence of these conditions was extracted retrospectively from the medical audit records for the three months before the study.

Patient workload

A recognised patient dependency tool, 'Criteria for Care', was used to determine whether the rostering of staff matched the dependency of the patients. This would allow conclusions about the current use of the nursing resource. The tool was adopted after staff training in its use and operated for a month. The data also enabled the calculation of bed occupancy over that period.

Patient throughput

The average length of stay over a three-month period before the study was calculated from the patient administration system. This was then compared to other hospitals' length of stay for the same patient group (gastrointestinal surgery).

Nursing records

The patient's nursing record should record the nursing practice on the ward. The quality of the documentation is vital to the quality of care and has been the subject of detailed audit in its own right (Phaneuf 1976). However, the Phaneuf Audit is long and complex, so key criteria were taken from it and adapted to enable an overview of the quality of the nursing records. The records of the 20 patients selected for interview were analysed.

Ward budget

The ward sister was responsible for the nursing staff budget. The cost of nurse staffing is the largest component of NHS expenditure and a significant factor in delivering a service within current resources. The relation of the ward expenditure on staffing to its base budget over the year was measured using data from the finance department.

Major conclusions

The audit suggested that the nurses were not identifying or meeting all the patients' needs. They felt overworked and frustrated about their personal contribution to patient care. Patients were receiving inadequate information about their course of treatment and how to manage after discharge. The nursing records suggested poor communication relating to patients' needs, with some potentially hazardous practices (not recording pre-operative checks). The workload was fairly predictable but the nursing resource was not matched to the patient demand. Bed capacity was underused and patient length of stay and post-operative complications were high. The latter would affect the former. The NDU was not operating efficiently or effectively. There were positive points in that the nursing team worked well together and supported each other and, on the whole, the patients did not feel dissatisfied with their care. It was these latter aspects that enabled the staff to agree on the key areas that needed addressing:

- Poor communication
- Underuse of all nurses' skills
- Lack of individual responsibility for patient care
- Poor discharge planning
- Poor pre-operative preparation to prevent post-operative complications
- Mismanagement of the nursing resource and bed capacity
- Lack of explicit standards to which staff could work
- Insufficient involvement of patients in the planning of their care

Changing the organisation and practice of nursing

The plan of change required the nurses on the NDU to choose solutions to these problems. The nursing development officer's role was to inform that choice and then to plan the pace of implementation, facilitating the change process. The sister decided that the most important way to influence the standard of care was by educating the staff and providing them with a framework for nursing practice which gave them job satisfaction. The current method of organising nursing care delivery was patient allocation. The method often claimed to give the most satisfaction was primary nursing (Manthey 1980), but this might take at least 18 months to introduce (Wright 1990). The staff were concerned that this should not be the only change and that it would not provide speedy results. Team (or modular) nursing was therefore chosen as the framework for care delivery (Kron 1981). The introduction of this new framework required negotiation with medical and other staff and support for the nurses as they began to take control of decision-making. The nursing staff took responsibility for producing patient information sheets for all the operations and procedures, in close liaison with medical staff. They also produced an information booklet about the ward, and a discharge booklet based on the work of Vaughan and Taylor (1988).

The ward duty rotas were to be analysed monthly to calculate staff supply and ensure it reflected the predicted pattern of demand. Recognising that the doctors tend to select the patients they bring in for surgery, the nurses agreed that the ward sister should liaise with the doctors to ensure a spread of workload. This also ensured that the easier cases were brought in during periods of staff shortfall and the more complex cases when the ward had its established staffing. There was also concern at the number of patients cancelled from the operating list after admission because they were unfit for surgery. To overcome this, and to begin pre-operative preparation as early as possible, the junior sister took responsibility for running a work-up clinic on the ward, using any spare bed capacity and the day room. It was anticipated that this close liaison with the doctors would enable better bed usage and a better match of staff skills to patient requirements.

It was decided to start from scratch and redesign the nursing record documentation to meet the new requirements. This included pilot stages. These records were then to be kept at the patient's bedside, for the use of both patients and nurses. This enabled access for both parties and ensured that patients were involved in planning their own care. Verbal handover from the nurses in the team to their colleagues on the next shift was also changed to involve the patients.

Finally, staff decided to write standards of care for those areas that had been of concern to patients – namely, admission, personal identity, patient awareness, pain, rest, safety and discharge. Staff involvement ensured ownership and the strategy for change included staff participation in regular meetings to overcome resistance. Staff education was vital and included workshops on the ward alongside visits to other sites and formal education programmes. Each staff member had her own personal development plan and performance review. Progress with each item was reviewed weekly and the pace of implementation altered accordingly. Ideas were encouraged and considered by the whole nursing team. There were inevitable mood swings and difficulties, but all these targets had been achieved after a year. One circuit of the audit cycle had been made and the ward was ready to be audited again.

The second audit

The second audit included one addition: the standards of care developed in the first year. The staff were apprehensive about the results: the ward had undergone significant changes in a relatively short time, and there was concern that these changes might not have had a chance to make a positive impact on the results. However, the results far exceeded expectations in staff and patient satisfaction and confirmed the areas that still required improvement. Over the year the nursing staff had managed to increase patient satisfaction dramatically, with areas of concern to patients shifting from poor nursing care to organisational matters outside the immediate control of the ward staff. This went hand in hand with an improvement in the quality of clinical care (clinical indicators) while improving efficiency (bed occupancy, length of stay, ward costs). Alongside this, staff morale had improved at a time when it was difficult to recruit and retain nursing staff in London.

The first year for the ward as an NDU was a pilot year in terms of determining viable and cost-effective changes in practice and steering this process through audit. It is noteworthy that costs had been reduced in nursing staffing (on the base budget and also on staff turnover costs), but also in other areas as a spin-off of reduced post-operative complications and improved discharge planning. As with the previous year, the audit required changes in practice and organisation of care. The ward had undergone one complete cycle of the audit, had undergone a second measurement and was planning the next developmental phases. The audit had led to developments in the practice and organisation of nursing on the ward, which had improved the value for money of the nursing service. The change strategy adopted had ensured that these developments were successful.

Conclusion

Evaluation enabled this NDU to plan change and to draw conclusions about the success of those changes. It provided results that were of interest to patients, nurses, doctors and general managers and demonstrated that investing in nursing reaps rewards for all. Evaluating your NDU will demonstrate the value of your work;

using evaluation in all aspects of your nursing ensures that the patient gets the best possible care.

References

Adelman C et al (1984) Rethinking Case Study. In J Ball et al. *Conducting Small Scale Investigations in Educational Management*. London: Harper & Row.

Hancock C (1990) Can it work for patients? *Senior Nurse* **10**(7): 8–10.

Humphries G and Turner A (1989) Job satisfaction and attitudes of nursing staff on a unit for the elderly infirm, with change of location. *Journal of Advanced Nursing* **14**: 298–307.

Kron T (1981) *The Management of Patient Care*, 5 edn. Philadelphia: W B Saunders.

Manthey M (1980) *The Practice of Primary Nursing*. Oxford: Blackwell Scientific Publications Inc.

Packwood T, Keen J and Buxton M (1991) *Hospitals in Transition: The Resource Management Experience*. Milton Keynes: Open University Press.

Patchen M (1970) *Achievement and Involvement on the Job*. Englewood Cliffs, NJ: Prentice Hall.

Pearson A, Durand I and Punton S (1989) Determining quality in a unit where nursing is the primary intervention. *Journal of Advanced Nursing* **14**: 269–273.

Phaneuf M (1976) *The Nursing Audit*. New York: Appleton-Century-Crofts.

Pollitt C (1984) Blunt tools: performance measurement in policies for health care. *International Journal of Management Science* **12**(2): 131–140.

Pollitt C (1986) A poor performance. *New Society* 3 October: 20–21.

Roberts H (1991) Measuring performance in the NHS. *Hospital Management International*: 94–104.

Salvage J (1990) Promoting good practice. *Nursing Standard* **4**(4): 52–3.

Stein L I, Watts D T and Howell T (1990) The doctor–nurse game revisited. *New England Journal of Medicine* **322**(8): 546–549.

Vaughan B and Taylor K (1988) Homeward Bound. *Nursing Times* **84**(15): 28–31.

Wright S (1990) *My Patient – My Nurse. The Practice of Primary Nursing*. London: Scutari Press.

Yin R (1984) *Case Study Research*. London: Sage.

NDUs – Just Another Bandwagon?

Jane Salvage and Stephen G Wright

What does the future hold for nursing development units? The number of NDUs has continued to expand since the first tentative steps in the early 1980s. In 1991, when further Department of Health monies were made available through the King's Fund Centre, 192 potential NDUs in a variety of settings put themselves forward for funding. They saw themselves as ready to take on the title of NDU. In addition, many other teams and units have adopted the title or have joined the King's Fund NDU network. Further work suggests that the number of NDUs continues to expand and that interest in becoming an NDU is still strong, both in the UK and overseas (Vaughan 1992, Wright 1992).

This growth is reinforced by encouragement in recent NHS documents, such as the NHS Management Executive objectives of 1993, which say there will be continued support for the spread of NDUs and the 'good practice' they encourage (Department of Health 1993). NDUs are part of the movement towards patient-centred change in nursing which Salvage (1992) described as the 'New Nursing'. This groundswell of innovation in nursing, of which NDUs are but one of many examples, is significant in one particular respect. NDUs are, by definition, practice-led. Management, education and research in health care can all contribute to change in nursing practice, but the NDU movement both symbolises and demonstrates the contribution of clinical nurses to the change process.

As with any innovation, the blossoming of NDUs has had its critics. There have been fears that NDUs will become another bandwagon which may be exploited by unsympathetic managers or will have their purpose and identity corrupted by misguided practitioners (Mangan 1992). There is perhaps some strength in the argument that nursing is prone to fashions which, for a time, are greeted with great debate, taken up enthusiastically and seen as panaceas. Much early work on nursing models, the nursing process and primary nursing would appear to support this view.

A number of people have proposed an accreditation system for NDUs in order to minimise some of these risks – in other words, to establish more rigid criteria for designation as an NDU. The King's Fund Centre has recently developed a peer group review system as well as refining its criteria for what can or cannot be designated an NDU. One regional health authority has set up its own accreditation scheme which identifies several categories of NDUs according to their stage of development (Malby 1992, Yorkshire Regional Health Authority 1992).

It is important to have some means of defining what an NDU is and is not, to avoid abusing or watering down the concept. At the same time, problems will arise if such schemes become excessively rigid or bureaucratic. One characteristic of NDUs has been their struggle to loosen the shackles of rigid systems in health care which stifle nursing creativity. It would be ironic if, in liberating themselves from one set of rules, they were to become constrained by another. The current accreditation schemes do not appear to have produced this negative effect, but the NDU movement must maintain its vigilance on this complex issue.

Another consequence of becoming an NDU is the charge of elitism. On the one hand, designation as an NDU can lead to greater organisational support, perhaps some additional funding and the legitimisation of the many changes which the NDU pursues. On the other hand, NDUs can be seen as 'tall poppies' (Faugier 1993): units, like individuals, which seek to innovate and stand out from the crowd may find recognition and support for their good work counterbalanced by hostility and criticism. Some nurses, and indeed some people in general, do not take kindly to others who seek to be different. Nurses in NDUs may have to cope with hostile colleagues who see the NDU as unfairly advantaged, or they may feel under great pressure to succeed in the public eye. Public exposure and willingness to struggle for best practice has its negative aspect (as illustrated by Black 1993 and Turner-Shaw and Bosanquet 1993).

Rule (1992) suggests that the difficulty many nurses have in celebrating and supporting success is an aspect of 'victim behaviour'. Feeling a sense of oppression, lack of support and exploitation as a group, nurses sometimes act out their anger and frustration on each other. This anger is more readily directed at those who are easily identified as 'different' – even more so if that difference highlights challenges and conflicts for every nurse's own practice. Thus, while NDUs have received much support and acclaim, they have also experienced varying degrees of reproach, deprecation and envy. As Mangan (1992) points out:

> To an extent they have become seen, perhaps unfairly, as elitist, and are perceived to have had more and more money, staff and general resources poured into them in order to ensure that they work.

The myth has arisen that NDUs are run by elite groups of nurses and have high levels of qualified staff and better funding. They are sometimes seen as centres of excellence where everything is perfect (Black 1993). This can produce difficulties for staff who feel that they constantly have to justify their work or deal with visitors who expect perfection but are quick to find fault.

These myths fly in the face of reality, as shown in recent research studies (notably Black 1993 and Turner-Shaw and Bosanquet 1993). In the new NHS structure, purchasers are writing into purchaser-provider contracts their wish to create more NDUs, but very few units receive additional funding; the majority, like the original Tameside NDU (Black 1993), have to work within existing budgets. Furthermore, there is no evidence to support the charge of 'elitist' NDUs and no indication from the existing literature that NDUs have laid claim to excellence or perfection, although they have made a commitment to aspire to these goals. Nor have NDUs tended to keep their work to themselves; indeed, it is one of their reasons for existence that their knowledge and research is readily shared with others by publishing, study days, visitors' programmes, and so on.

The difficulties described here are often, perhaps inevitably, confronted in any setting where there is a commitment to change. Part of the work of NDUs is to manage change systematically, taking account of these factors. In so doing they stimulate the development of change mastery and clinical leadership. Through their outcomes – in terms of the effects on care and the nurses who give it – the impact of the NDU goes way beyond the original pilot site. The work of the NDU is ultimately transmitted elsewhere (a commitment to do so is one of its characteristic features). Practice is changed in parallel with the people who deliver it. Thus there is movement from 'a unit capable of fragmented innovation' into 'not only a nursing development unit but a *person* development unit

enhancing the quality of life of all who encounter its influence'
(Lewis 1991).

NDUs in the UK now number several hundred. As a result of the
work of the World Health Organisation and The European Nursing
Development Agency, among others, similar schemes are now
emerging elsewhere in Europe, with exciting beginnings in clinical
practice development taking place in the countries of Central and
Eastern Europe as well as the European Union. What started off as
a small local issue has emerged as a phenomenon of national and
international significance for nursing and health care. There are
many ways of producing innovation in nursing, but for good or ill
the NDU bandwagon is now rolling. While it is unlikely that all
nursing settings can or will be NDUs, perhaps the NDU movement
will have achieved its goals when the principles and practices it
espouses have become more universally adopted. Even then, there
will always be a need for centres which expand and research the
boundaries of nursing. When health services are going through
difficult and uncertain times, NDUs may be candles in the dark,
preserving and developing nursing's humanitarian values and
practice. Despite the current problems of the NHS and other health
care systems, with their emphasis on money and crude productivity
standing in opposition to altruism, equity and quality, innovative
nursing practice can still flourish.

The evaluation of the impact and outcomes of NDUs on people's
health will be an important factor in their future. Evidence is
already beginning to emerge that developing nurses and nursing,
supporting innovation and creating a climate for best practice
through NDUs has positive benefits not only for nurses but also for
the quality of patient care. The link between better quality of care,
increased cost-effectiveness and the development of qualified nurses
is now being demonstrated – a trend that may continue as more
results emerge from the many NDU research programmes and
projects.

NDUs are part of the movement for change in nursing; this book
has argued that they are one of its flagships. They are not an end in
themselves, but part of a continuous process of innovation. When
the power and potential of nursing practice is liberated in this way,
they can have a direct impact on health for all. This, in the end, is the
purpose of the NDU – to transform nurses and nursing in order to
help improve people's health. We hope the ideas and experiences
collected in this book will contribute to that goal.

References

Black M (1993) *The Growth of the Tameside Nursing Development Unit.* London: King's Fund Centre.

Department of Health (1993) *Management Executive Business Plan for 1993/4.* Leeds: NHSME.

Faugier J (1993) Tall poppies. *Nursing Times* **88**(50): 20.

Lewis D (1991) *Primary Nursing at St Luke's Hospital.* Unpublished paper. Huddersfield: St Luke's Nursing Development Unit.

Malby R (1992) Accredit where it's due. *Nursing Times* **88**(43): 48–50.

Mangan P (1992) Where from here? *Nursing Times* **88**(50): 34–35.

Rule J (1992) *Nurses as Victims.* Paper given at RCN Congress, Harrogate (unpublished).

Salvage J (1992) The New Nursing: Empowering Patients or Empowering Nurses? In J Robinson et al (eds) *Policy Issues in Nursing.* Milton Keynes: Open University Press.

Turner-Shaw J and Bosanquet N (1993) *A Way to Develop Nurses and Nursing.* London: King's Fund Centre.

Vaughan B (1992) The pursuit of excellence. *Nursing Times* **88**(31): 26–28.

Wright S G (1992) Exporting Excellence. *Nursing Times* **88**(39): 40–42.

Yorkshire Regional Health Authority (1992) *Nursing Development Unit Accreditation Scheme.* Harrogate: YRHA.

Select Bibliography

This list contains the editor's selection of some of the key texts which discuss issues central to nursing development. Other references can be found at the end of each chapter.

Audit Commission (1992) *Making Time for Patients: A Handbook for Ward Sisters*. London: HMSO.
Beardshaw V and Robinson R (1990) *New for Old? Prospects for Nursing in the 1990s*. King's Fund Institute Research Report 8. London: King's Fund.
Benner P (1984) *From Novice to Expert*. Menlo Park, CA: Addison-Wesley.
Black G (ed.) (1992) *Nursing Development Units: Work in Progress*. London: King's Fund Centre.
Hawkins P and Shohet R (1989) *Supervision in the Helping Professions*. Milton Keynes: Open University Press.
Manthey M (1980) *The Practice of Primary Nursing*. Boston, MA: Blackwell Scientific.
Pearson A (1983) *The Clinical Nursing Unit*. London: Heinemann.
Pearson A (1992) *Nursing at Burford – A Story of Change*. London: Scutari Press.
Pearson A and Vaughan B (1986) *Nursing Models for Practice*. London: Heinemann.
Pearson A, Punton S and Durand I (1992) *Nursing Beds – An Evaluation of Therapeutic Nursing*. London: Scutari Press.
Pembrey S (1989) The development of nursing practice: A new contribution. *Senior Nurse* 9(8): 3–8.
Salvage J (1985) *The Politics of Nursing*. London: Heinemann.
Salvage J (1991) Making the best use of nursing skills: managers and clinicians in partnership. *Journal of Management in Medicine* 5(1): 54–59.
Salvage J (1992) The New Nursing: Empowering Patients or Empowering Nurses? In J Robinson, A Gray and R Elkan (eds) *Policy Issues in Nursing*. Milton Keynes: Open University Press.
Salvage J (ed.) (1993) *Nursing in Action: Strengthening Nursing and Midwifery to Support Health for All*. World Health Organization, European Series 48,

Copenhagen.

Stocking B (1985) *Initiative and Inertia: Case Studies in the NHS*. London: Nuffield Provincial Hospitals Trust.

Towell D and Harries C (eds) 1979) *Innovation in Patient Care*. London: Croom Helm.

Walton M (1982) *Management and Managing: A Dynamic Approach*. Lippincott Nursing Series. London: Harper & Row.

Wright S (1989) *Changing Nursing Practice*. London: Edward Arnold.

Wright S (1990) *Building and Using A Model of Nursing*, 2nd edn. London: Edward Arnold.

Wright S (1990) *My Patient – My Nurse*. London: Scutari Press.

APPENDIX I

Selection Criteria Used to Assess and Guide Applicants for Department of Health NDU Grants, 1992. Drawn up by the Nursing Developments Programme, King's Fund Centre.

In order to ensure equal opportunities the following criteria have been identified to be used in the selection of units for allocation of grants. It is recognised that each unit may be at a different stage of development in relationship to each of these issues. However, success is more likely if evidence can be shown of consideration of them all. The order does not indicate priority and need not be adhered to in applications:

1. *Development of Nursing.* The development of nursing is central to the work of an NDU and a clear statement of the way in which this will be achieved is essential. Evidence is needed of the vision towards which the unit is working, together with a focused strategy which outlines how this progress will be made. This may include: – an outline of the philosophy and values held by the unit staff; – a clearly expressed core purpose of the development work, including a statement of the aims and expected outcomes; – an outline plan of the way in which these outcomes may be achieved, including a tentative time scale; – an indication of who will be involved with, and take responsibility for different aspects of the project; – a justification of the priorities within the project in meeting both professional and organisational goals.

Both small- and large-scale development can bring benefits to patients and their families and are of equal importance to the whole project.

2. *Clinical Leadership.* Successful and lasting change depends largely on the presence of strong clinical leadership. It is therefore important that a clinical leader who has day-to-day responsibility for the delivery of nursing care can be identified. It is also helpful to know whether this is the person who will act as the major change agent, with responsibility for the progress of the project.

3. *Commitment from the Organisation.* No change can take place in isolation and it is important to establish the place of an NDU within the wider organisation. To this end it is helpful to establish a steering group who can assist in reviewing activities, disseminating information about the purpose and work of the NDU and offering support and guidance.

Similarly it is important that there is an organisational climate which is conducive to change, showing openness, trust, effective communication and freedom from inappropriate constraints.

The impact of an NDU can and should be wide-reaching both within and beyond nursing. Thus evidence of the support and commitment from senior nurses in managerial or educational roles, medical and paramedical colleagues, unit general managers or chief executives and members of the health authority is advisable.

The purchaser-provider scenario also needs to be given consideration. The role of an NDU as the provider of service and the interest of the purchaser in future commissioning of these services needs to be addressed. Any changes which have implications in relationship to the provision of a specific service need to be considered.

4. *Staff Participation.* It is vital that all unit staff are encouraged to take ownership of the project from the outset in order that the whole team becomes committed to its success. The manner in which they have been or will be involved should be clearly identified. A profile of the current and/ or future clinical nursing team involved in the project may be helpful. Where new roles are being developed thought should be given to lines of responsibility and accountability.

5. *Staff Development.* An important aspect of any development work is the growth of the staff themselves as well as of the service. Indeed, empowerment of nurses is seen as one way through which patients may be empowered. This may entail the provision of both formal and informal learning opportunities, as well as the provision of personal support. There may be resource implications other than direct financing such as availability of time and facilities. Evidence of the way in which these needs can be met needs to be given consideration, bearing in mind that continuing education need not always take place in a formal arena.

6. *Evaluation.* While all people involved in the delivery of a health care service are concerned with improvements in quality, different groups may have specific interests in different aspects. Thus when planning evaluation strategies it may be helpful to consider who will be interested in the outcomes of the project. In this way criteria can be identified which would be pertinent to a wider audience. For example, cost-effectiveness is evidently of concern to those with managerial responsibilities, while changes in clinical outcomes may be more pertinent to professional health care workers.

As a general principle it is helpful to use more than one approach to evaluation and where appropriate to take advantage of the wide number of tools which are already available. Collecting baseline data (how things are now) and measuring progress over time can reassure the NDU team and provide vital evidence of change as well as pointers for future development.

There is a great emphasis being placed on the importance of 'outcome measures' in the current health care climate and wherever possible information of this type would be very helpful.

7. *Finance.* Evidence will be sought of current and continuing commitment by the health authority/Trust board for providing adequate resources for the unit. Costing for the use of additional resources which may be grant funded should also be produced. It is helpful if these are broken down under sub-headings, such as salaries, equipment, educational development, clerical, consumables. Predicted changes in local financial arrangements should be outlined and implications for the NDU considered. We would recommend that inflation is costed at a 10 per cent rise for years 2 and 3 to allow a safe margin.

8. *Equal Opportunities.* The King's Fund Centre is committed to equal opportunities for staff and users of health services and some evidence of how this is being addressed within the unit would be appropriate.

APPENDIX II

Guidelines for the Use of a Nursing Development Unit Bursary

(Example from Tameside NDU)

1. The general aim of the bursary is to assist nurses with defraying the costs of their continued professional education.
2. The funds given to and arising from the bursary are used exclusively for the development and support of nursing staff in the Nursing Development Unit (Care of the Elderly).
3. The funding of the bursary is derived primarily from the work of the consultant nurse and the fund raising committee in creating links and sponsorship with the local community and industry, and other income-generating measures such as:

   • Profits arising from conferences, courses and seminars
   • Visitors' fees and donations
   • Sale of copies of nursing documentation and research papers
   • Interest on money invested in the bursary

4. Funding from the bursary is open to all non-student nurses within the Nursing Development Unit (Care of the Elderly).
5. A nurse seeking funds will set out details of the request in writing and submit it to the consultant nurse. Details required include:

   (a) The nature of the course of study/research project to be completed
   (b) The costs to be incurred
   (c) Details of any project work to be completed
   (d) The purpose of the course of study/research project

6. Funds are awarded after consideration by the consultant nurse, liaising as necessary with the senior nurse manager, the unit accountant and general manager.
7. Nurses receiving awards are expected to remain in the employment of the Nursing Development Unit for at least 12 months after the completion

of their course. A signed undertaking to this effect may be requested.

8. Candidates for funding may be requested to present themselves for interview to the bursary committee comprised of members as at (6) above. The panel's decision on an award of funding is final.

9. Day-to-day monitoring of expenditure, balances, etc. in the bursary will be carried out by the unit accountant.

10. Nurses awarded funding will normally be paid by cheque, after request by the consultant nurse to the treasurer's department.

11. No withdrawals can be made from the bursary without the expressed consent of the consultant nurse or in his/her absence, the senior nurse manager for the Nursing Development Unit.

12. A summary of the use of the bursary will be included in the Nursing Development Unit's Annual Report.

13. Awards from the bursary are made to defray the cost of items such as course fees, travel expenses, project typing and other expenses as deemed appropriate. Funds to defray such costs may be awarded in whole or in part, at the discretion of the consultant nurse and/or the bursary committee.

14. The Nursing Development Unit bursary is also used to provide funds to purchase textbooks and pay for journal subscriptions for the NDU library.

15. The bursary may also be used to support the cost of secretarial/research assistance for the NDU as may be necessary from time to time.

16. The bursary is also used to underwrite the cost of conferences arranged on behalf of the NDU, although it is expected that all such conferences are organised on a profit-making or break-even basis.

17. In the event of the failure to complete a course/research project, then any funds awarded may be required to be repaid to the NDU. The nurse will be required to sign an undertaking to this effect. Exceptions to this rule may be granted at the discretion of the consultant nurse and/or the bursary committee after submission of relevant facts to them.

18. Any nurse accepting an award from the bursary must be prepared to:
    (a) Provide a written summary of the course/project to the bursary awards committee on completion
    (b) Submit details of the project to professional journals if considered suitable for publication
    (c) Remain in employment of the Nursing Development Unit area for at least one year afterwards
    (d) Make an oral presentation to colleagues on the outcome of the project where appropriate

19. The bursary is concerned solely with the award of funding: time off to attend the courses is not necessarily guaranteed, although applications

will be viewed sympathetically. Request for study time must be made in the usual way through the senior nurse manager.

20. Copies of this policy will be made available to all nursing settings in the Nursing Development Unit.

21. Advice and support on the submission of funding requests and the completion and writing up of projects can be obtained from the consultant nurse.

APPENDIX IIIa

Guidance on the International Exchange Programme

(Example from Tameside NDU)

The international exchange idea began in 1985 with two nurses, Barbara Reed from Emory University Hospital, Atlanta, and Steve Wright from the Tameside Nursing Development Unit. These nurses visited each other's country and returned home filled with ideas.

Setting up a system to make it easier for staff to exchange countries began, their ideas brought together by colleagues. Letters crossed the Atlantic and two quite different cultures and health care systems built a foundation of a programme that was to follow.

Nurses would be exchanged between the twinned health settings of Emory University Hospital and Wesley Woods Geriatric Hospice, Atlanta, Georgia, and the Nursing Development Unit, Tameside and Glossop Health Authority, Ashton-under-Lyne. The focus would be on the care of elderly people.

Many potential benefits lay ahead. Not only could nurses learn and share in a general sense about nursing in another country, but they could also contribute to international understanding. The more people meet from different cultures, the better they can understand one another, both as citizens and nurses.

The exchange programme between Atlanta and Tameside grew and now incorporates hospitals in Germany, London, Glasgow and Russia. Obviously, language can be a barrier in some countries and this must be taken into account when exchanges take place. All persons participating have clearly set objectives beforehand, with statements of work to be completed on return.

Within all of this, the nurses also have an opportunity to enjoy themselves, taking pleasure in visiting another country and meeting new people – something that is denied to many.

Motivated and invigorated, nurses return in a better position to enhance their contribution to their place of work and to the care of their patients.

APPENDIX IIIb

Tameside NDU – International Exchange Guidelines

There is a diverse and rich body of knowledge in nursing in both countries and there is much that the two groups of nurses can learn from each other. Each group of nurses is beset by problems which have much more in common. They are making innovations and exploring new territory, often quite ignorant of each other's work and potentially wasting much effort in reinventing the wheel. The main aims of the exchange system may be summarised thus:

1. The purpose of international exchange is to set up a 'twinning system' between Tameside and an overseas health care setting.
2. A link person in each setting will act as overall coordinator of the scheme. At Tameside, this will be the consultant nurse in the nursing development unit.
3. Each coordinator will exchange written information in nursing developments in their respective countries and disseminate this to appropriate nurses in their places of work and through their professional activities and organisations.
4. Each coordinator will provide addresses for staff with common interests to 'network' and exchange views and information directly through correspondence.
5. A list of contact persons will be drawn up to identify people in both settings who are willing to provide information, both in writing and through direct contact, by means of exchange visits. This will include those willing to offer hospitality and accommodation, to keep costs to a minimum.
6. The coordinators will also assist in the acquisition of funds to support the exchange of staff between the countries and devise suitable strategies for selecting appropriate staff to make the exchanges. At Tameside the Nursing Development Unit bursary will be used.
7. The coordinator will seek other potential sources of accommodation or hospitality and provide the respective traveller with guidance on travel

and cultural matters related to such exchanges.

8. Exchanges will take three main forms as judged appropriate by the senior nursing, clinical and management staff concerned:

    (a) Exchange of written information on current and proposed practices, for example, in such fields as innovative clinical nursing techniques, educational developments, quality assurance, and so on. There appears to be an enormous range of suitable topics which fit this category.

    (b) Exchange of nurses for short study visits, perhaps two or three weeks where specific issues are to be pursued in depth. The hospital in the country of origin will provide the funding to get the visitor there, while it is expected that the receiving country will seek to provide hospitality and accommodation at minimal cost. Staff making such visits will be expected to produce detailed reports of their study on return to circulate to both health authorities and to be reviewed for publication in the nursing press.

    (c) Exchange visits of a longer period – perhaps three to six months, where selected staff will simultaneously 'swap' jobs for this time and work in each other's settings. Support arrangements will apply as (b) above. Written reports will be prepared during and after the visit and submitted as agreed beforehand.

9. All persons participating in these exchanges will have clearly set objectives beforehand, with statements of work to be completed and other requirements. Serious attention must be paid to the dissemination of the knowledge gained to relevant persons, both inside and outside the appropriate health authorities, and to the nursing press for wider publication.

10. While initially being nursing-led, it is recognised that a variety of staff in each health system will gain much from a similar system of exchanging of people and information. It is anticipated, therefore, that the exchange system will eventually develop a multi-disciplinary nature with an opportunity for others in the health care team to participate and benefit from the system on similar guidelines.

Application details

1. The Nursing Development Unit bursary will fund the essential costs of the overseas trip including accommodation and transport and a contribution towards 'pocket money'.
2. The length of stay is usually two weeks.
3. Study leave will be granted through the nurse managers.
4. The applicants must:
   (a) Submit a proposal for an aspect of nursing the elderly which they would like to study overseas
   (b) Complete the study in writing and submit it to the consultant nurse
5. The applicant must be prepared to remain an employee of the Care of the Elderly Unit for at least 12 months after the completion of the study tour.
6. All transport and accommodation arrangements will be made for the applicant.
7. The proposal should contain:
   (a) The title of the project
   (b) Full details of the project (attaching supplementary information if necessary)
   (c) The reasons for choosing this subject
   (d) The benefits to be derived from the study
   (e) The benefits which the applicant hopes to bring to the patients and staff on the unit as a result of the visit
8. The applicant's personal details and those of the proposed study topics should be submitted with a covering letter (see form).

The consultant nurse will assist in clarification on any points if needed.

APPENDIX IV

Useful Addresses

Nursing Developments Programme,
King's Fund Centre for Health Services Development,
126 Albert Street,
London NW1 7NF
Telephone 0171–267 6111; Fax 0171–267 6108

Services include a Nursing Developments Network, established to facilitate the dissemination of ideas and sharing of experience in relation to nursing, midwifery and health visiting development. Membership, open to units and individuals, offers a newsletter, bibliographies, conferences and workshops and information exchange.

Nursing and Midwifery Unit,
Regional Office for Europe,
World Health Organisation,
Scherfigsvej 8,
2100 Copenhagen Ø
Denmark
Fax (+45) 39 17 18 65

The unit's current priority is support for nursing and midwifery development in the countries of Central and Eastern Europe and the former Soviet Union. Activities include encouraging the establishment of clinical development projects, publications, national and international meetings of nursing leaders and production of a basic package of learning materials on nursing (the LEMON project).

The European Nursing Development Agency (TENDA),
Tameside General Hospital,
Fountain Street,
Ashton-under-Lyne,
Lancashire OL5 9RW
Telephone 0161–339 5535; Fax 0161–339 5512

TENDA was set up to continue the consultancy and development work originating in the Tameside NDU. By providing courses and workshops and consultancy in the TENDA facilities and on site in local health organisations, TENDA supports the development of nurses and nursing. TENDA actively raises funds to support this work and has created and used its own charitable funds. Many projects are under way in the UK and throughout Europe.

Index